T0143819

BASIC HEALTH PUBLICATIONS USER'S GUIDE

TO PREVENTING & TREATING HEADACHES NATURALLY

Learn How You Can Use Diet and Supplements to Put an End to Headaches.

JONATHAN M. BERKOWITZ, M.D.

JACK CHALLEM Series Editor

Series Editor: Jack Challem
Editor: Susan Andrews
Typesetter: Gary A. Rosenberg
Series Cover Designer: Mike Stromberg

Basic Health Publications User's Guides are published by Basic Health Publications, Inc.

CONTENTS

INTRODUCTION

Raise your hand if you've never had a head-ache. Well, I guess if you're reading this book, you probably have had more than your share of headaches. My point, however, is that I'd expect to see very few hands in the air. If misery loves company, people with headaches certainly have plenty of company. Indeed, it is no secret that at least 90 percent of the population experience at least one headache yearly. This book is not for the individual who has one headache a year. Rather, this book is for those unfortunate people whose headaches profoundly affect their lives. This book is for those 40 percent of the population who will tell you that their headaches are severe and de-bilitating. It's for those people whose headaches present a weekly or almost daily battle to lead a normal life. Although headaches may substanti-ally disrupt a person's life, the good news is that for most people, the vast majority of headaches are benign and temporary, and do not portend a more serious disorder.

Perhaps the most important things to under-stand about headaches are why they occur and what can be done to treat and prevent them: the essential purpose of this book. An even more im-portant purpose of this book is to help you not only to identify and remove potential headache triggers from your life, but also to give you the natural means of successfully treating headaches when they occur.

Chapter 1 is devoted to describing headaches

and identifying which symptoms represent the typical headache versus which symptoms demand more serious medical attention. Also included in Chapter 1 are descriptions of how diet and emotions add to the headache equation. In Chapter 2, you'll learn about the basic headache syndromes, such as migraine, tension, and cluster headaches. Chapter 3 is devoted to vitamin, mineral, and herbal headache supplements and the studies that support their use, and Chapter 4 describes several alternative headache therapies that have been successfully used, such as exercise, acupuncture, and biofeedback. Finally, Chapter 5 describes the basic pharmacologic management of headache, the treatment of last resort.

WHAT IS A HEADACHE?

At its simplest level, a headache represents head pain. We normally think of pain as resulting from an injury to a bodily site; the sensation is then transmitted through nerves to the brain and is perceived as pain. For headache sufferers, this scenario is only true in relatively rare conditions that involve facial nerves like the trigeminal nerve, a major nerve that transmits sensations from the face to the brain. It may surprise many of you to learn that most parts of the brain and head do not feel pain and only the scalp, dural sinuses, and blood vessels can actually perceive pain. The dural sinuses are like large veins in the head that carry blood away from the brain. While researchers are still sorting out where headache pain really comes from, scientists suspect that some headaches originate from deep inside the brain, in a region called the midbrain.

Headache
A generic term that relates to pain anywhere in the head, including the face. There are many types and causes of headache.

Nonetheless, there are only a few structures within the skull that can actually feel pain. As mentioned, some of the head's arteries and veins can feel pain, and we know that pain occurs when these vessels are distended, inflamed, or pulled on. The same goes for cranial nerves that can transmit pain from the face or send pain signals to the brain when they themselves are injured or inflamed. Another head-pain mechanism originates in the meningies, the tough sheet-like structure that covers the brain. Pain results when the meningies are inflamed or compressed. A classic cause of meningeal irritation is seen in meningitis, an infection of the meningies caused by bacteria.

Meningies
Tough fiberlike covering of the brain that can rarely get infected and inflamed, such as in meningitis.

Obviously, the most common headache symptom is pain. This pain can be localized to a specific area of the head or can be generalized. Although pain may be the most common symptom, many headaches are accompanied by other symptoms, such as fatigue, visual changes, nausea, and vomiting. Indeed, one of the most common types of headaches is the migraine, whose classical symptoms include throbbing head pain, visual disturbances, and nausea with or without vomiting. Although headaches can display a variety of symptoms, different types of headaches often present typical symptoms. I will discuss these headaches and how they present in more detail later. For now, let's review some of the general diagnostic features of headache.

The course and duration of headache pain can be helpful in diagnosing its cause. For instance, in a common tension headache, the head pain builds gradually over a course of minutes to hours. Migraine pain develops over a period of hours, can last from hours to days, and tends to get better with sleep. Conversely, the pain associated with a ruptured aneurysm often strikes like a lightning bolt. An aneurysm is an abnormally formed and thinned portion of a blood vessel that can rupture without warning. Some people are born with aneurysms while other aneurysms can be caused by disease.

Most commonly, headache location is vague and does not accurately correspond to where the head pain originates. However, in headaches caused by inflammatory disorders, such as arteritis, the patient can very accurately pinpoint the source of his or her pain. Indeed, in arteritis, the pain is normally localized right over the diseased vessel. Sinus or dental pain also produces discomfort in a relatively small area.

Diagnosing Headaches

As you probably know, it does not take a rocket scientist to tell you that you have a headache. It does, however, take some effort and thought to discover what type of headache you have. Perhaps one of the most important clues to the seriousness of a disorder is how long the symptoms have lasted. For instance, someone who walks into my office with their first-ever headache raises more red flags than a person who complains about the same type of head pain for thirty years. In other words, the more recent the symptoms, the more potential for a serious underlying disorder.

When being seen by a physician for headaches, you should expect to provide a complete history and physical, and to receive a neurological exam, of which the physician will take particular note. You may also need a computed tomography (CT scan) or a magnetic resonance imaging (MRI) study of your head to make sure nothing serious is wrong. As some headaches are caused by hypertension, expect to have your blood pressure checked. Also insist that your eyes be checked for glaucoma, an occasional cause of head pain.

When Is a Headache Not a Headache?

Not all headaches are created equal. Although the vast majority of headaches result either from tension or migraine-type head pain, there are several other conditions that can cause headache. The simple viral infection is one of the most common of these conditions. Virtually every person on Earth can attest to the fact that when ill with a cold or flu they have had a headache. These headaches, however, are a temporary annoyance and normally resolve when the illness clears up. Other, more serious medical conditions that are typically accompanied by headache include lupus, infectious mononucleosis, and inflammatory bowel disease. These headaches tend to be recurrent and chronic and are associated with the underlying disease activity. Contrary to popular belief, high blood pressure is a rare cause of headache, and it normally takes very high blood pressure readings to cause head pain. Nevertheless, hypertension is a silent killer of men and women and every person should have their blood pressure checked regularly. Other uncommon causes of headache include drugs, such as birth control pills.

People also get headaches from sinusitis or glaucoma. Facial pain usually originates from structures located in the face or sinus. For instance, throbbing pain that occurs either above or below the eye, and close to the nose, is often sinus related. Likewise, tooth pain can be found anywhere along the jaw, the maxilla, or the ear. Sometimes the facial nerves become diseased and produce sharp and sudden electric shocklike pain. Known as "neuralgias," nerve disease can cause some of the most excruciating facial pain. Most of the time, neuralgia pain occurs without warning; however, this type of pain can also be precipitated by chewing. Pain with chewing can also be caused by temporomandibular joint dysfunction (TMJ), arteritis, or tooth disease. Undoubtedly, dental pain is by far the most common type of facial pain; it can be felt almost anywhere in the face and is often precipitated by eating, especially hot or cold foods or flu-

Neuralgia

A generic term referring to a diseased nerve that can result in head pain. The prototypical neuralgia is trigeminal neuralgia, a disease of the trigeminal nerve that often causes severe facial pain.

ids. Head pain related to glaucoma is often referred to the eye and may be accompanied by nausea and vomiting

Mercifully, the vast majority of headaches are nothing more than a nuisance. As we have seen, however, some headaches can indicate more serious disease. Whenever a healthcare professional is confronted with a complaint of headache, he or she must first rule out serious disease prior to labeling the condition "tension headache" or "migraine."

Of the several serious but fortunately rare causes of headache, the most important ones to consider are brain tumor, meningitis, arteritis, and subarachnoid hemorrhage (brain bleed). Although these conditions are rare, because of their serious nature, I will consider each separately.

Sometimes head pain is related to a diseased blood vessel, the classic example being temporal or giant cell arteritis. This rare condition represents a painful inflammatory disorder of the temporal artery. Usually occurring in the seventh decade of life, the disorder affects women more than men. The classic symptoms of arteritis include fever, headache, body aches, weight loss, and jaw pain when eating. It is important to diagnose arteritis early since about half of those who do not receive appropriate treatment go blind. While approximately 50 percent of those afflicted have pain in the temporal region, the head pain can occur anywhere. Unlike a migraine where the pain is vaguely described as being "deep" within the brain, many people with arteritis can tell exactly where their pain lies on the skull. Indeed, in temporal arteritis, the scalp pain may be so severe that even the lightest touch results in

Subarachnoid Bleeding

Bleeding in the head usually caused by the rupture of a small blood vessel covering the brain. It usually causes immediate and intense head pain, and can be fatal.

extreme pain. Occasionally there is redness over the inflamed artery accompanied by a tender nodule. While temporal arteritis is a serious disorder that if left untreated can cause blindness, the disease responds rapidly to medications making prompt medical attention vital.

Another rare cause of head pain is a tumor. If you tend to be a bit paranoid like me, every time you have a headache you're almost sure it's a brain tumor. Mercifully, the vast majority of headaches are harmless and brain tumors are exceedingly rare. Danger signs that head pain may be tumor related include headaches that begin in the early morning and improve during the day. Another warning sign are headaches that wake an individual from their sleep, a feature reported in about 10 percent of those with brain tumors. Vomiting is another worrisome sign, especially when it occurs several days to weeks prior to the start of headache. Many brain tumors, however, produce no head pain at all and only become apparent when they are well advanced. When tumors do cause head pain, the pain usually comes and goes and is moderate in severity. Brain tumor–related pain tends to be a dull aching pain that feels as if it is coming from deep within the brain. The pain is often made worse by maneuvers, such as lifting, coughing, or bending.

A condition that often mimics the symptoms of brain tumor is pseudotumor cerebri. This is an uncommon malady caused by elevated intracranial pressure with the typical victim being a young female who is often obese. Besides suffering from headaches, these individuals can also have visual disturbances, such as blind spots.

From a physician's perspective, the brain tumor signs of greatest concern are cranial nerve deficits. Cranial nerves arise from the brain stem and usually control functions above the neck, such as pupillary dilatation or hearing. Another warning sign that something more serious may be occurring is increasing headache frequency in someone who has rarely been troubled by headache.

Meningitis is another serious cause of headache. Although we've all heard about this potentially deadly infection of the brain's covering, meningitis is mercifully a medical rarity. Nevertheless, given the potential lethality of this disease, you should know some of its most prominent symptoms. The typical meningitis patient complains of a stiff neck with a severe headache and fever. If you or someone you know has fever or a stiff neck associated with headache, they should go immediately to the nearest emergency room to be evaluated. Although meningitis is a serious, life-threatening disorder, it can normally be successfully treated with antibiotics.

Severe headache with neck stiffness can also be seen during a brain bleed. Bleeding into the head or brain can occur for a variety of disorders, such as stroke or a ruptured aneurysm. A ruptured aneurysm can be accompanied by head pain and neck stiffness without fever, whereas stroke victims usually display other symptoms, such as limb (arm or leg) weakness and paralysis (or both).

Headache Warning Signs

So, how do you tell a "benign" headache from one that represents a more serious disorder? Without a doubt, headaches are a challenge to physicians to diagnose, given the variety of headache types as well as the variability of symptoms. In general, physicians consider the quality, location, and time course to be some of the most critical variables. Also important are the actions that make the symptoms better or worse. You may be surprised to learn that symptom intensity rarely offers any insight as to the cause of the headache. People can have totally "benign" but excruciating headache pain but lead an otherwise entirely normal life. Conversely, many people with a brain tumor have only mild symptoms or no symptoms at all. Also high on the list of warning signs are headaches or facial pain that are associated with a loss of facial sensation.

Aiding the diagnosis of headache is the knowledge that many headache syndromes follow predictable patterns. For instance, your typical tension headache is normally described as a tight band-like aching pain that feels like it is coming from deep inside the skull. Although the vast majority of headaches ultimately turn out to be harmless, several warning signs that may signal a more serious disorder are listed below:

- Vomiting prior to headache

- First-ever severe headache

- Fever with headache

- Headache wakes patient up from sleep

- Headache appears right after waking

- Headache that results from lifting, coughing, or bending

- New headache that occurs after age fifty-five

- Headache that gets worse over a period of days to weeks

- Headache described as "worst" ever

- Headache associated with neurological deficits

Diet and Headaches

It should not be surprising that many people blame certain foods for causing their headaches. Without a doubt, headache can be a manifestation of food sensitivity or allergy and we know that many people with migraine can identify certain foods as triggers. According to one study published in *The Lancet*, 66 percent of those with severe migraine had food allergies. The list of potential foods and additives that are associated with headache is extensive. For instance, the protein tryptophan has been implicated in migraine headaches, an observation that was demonstrated by one group of researchers who placed ten women with migraines on a tryptophan-restricted diet. Not surprisingly, the participants reported reduced migraine symptoms with tryptophan restriction. Likewise, the artificial sweetener aspartame has received considerable attention as a headache trigger. One study from the Montefiore Medical Center in New York City examined the role of diet in headache and found that 8.3 percent of participants identified aspartame as a trigger. In a similar vein, alcohol was blamed by 49.7 percent of participants as being a headache trigger. While the following list is far from complete, it represents the major food and additive triggers:

- Amines
- Aspartame
- Caffeine
- Chocolate
- Hypoglycemia
- Ice cream

- Lactose intolerance
- L-tryptophan
- MSG (monosodium glutamate)
- Nitrates
- Salt
- Sugar, refined

Given the fact that food allergies and sensitivities play an important role in headache, especially migraines, it is not surprising that multiple studies have shown that certain diets can help people with headache.

A high intake of carbohydrate leads to elevated serotonin, and several researchers have noted that carbohydrate-rich diets can help people with migraines. For instance, one group of scientists placed seven patients with

Serotonin
A neurotransmitter that plays a role in mood, sleep, pain, and sexual behavior. Serotonin dysfunction has been found in headache syndromes.

migraine on a low protein–tryptophan, high-carbohydrate diet. Improved symptoms were noted in the classic migraine group; however, no significant improvement was seen in the common migraine patients. According to the authors, "the apparent positive effect in the classic migraineurs could be due to a reduced intake of migraine-precipitating foods and/or increased brain serotonin levels."

In another study from Israel, researchers reported "marked clinical alleviation" in lactase-deficient migraine patients who were given a milk protein–free diet.

Given these considerations, if you suffer from headaches, a complete nutritional evaluation by someone who is experienced in diet and headache is clearly warranted.

What is especially helpful is the maintenance of a food-headache diary. This is simply a listing a foods you eat daily with a log of headache symptoms. What you may discover is that your headaches tend to occur after you eat certain foods. Once such observations are made, the food can be withdrawn from your diet and the frequency of symptoms again observed. Then, the food can be reintroduced into the diet with similar observations made on headache symptoms. Through a process of elimination, many people find that certain foods make their headaches worse whereas other foods improve them. Of course, it is highly recommended that you locate a healthcare professional experienced in nutritional evaluation, as his or her assistance will be especially valuable in pursuing this process.

CHAPTER 2

THE A-TO-Z GUIDE TO HEADACHES

The International Headache Society Classification of Headache lists more than sixty different types of headaches. Mercifully, we are only going to review the most common types that afflict most people.

Cluster Headache

Cluster headaches are a vascular type of headache that is characterized by brief but intense periods of pain, and that occurs above or below the eyes. Most of these attacks are short-lived but can occur frequently, up to three times daily for one to two months. This disorder is found in men more frequently than in women and tends to occur either chronically or episodically, with most cluster headaches occurring in a regular or circadian pattern. Attacks are commonly characterized by intense nighttime pain.

The most dramatic feature of a cluster headache is the pain, which is often sharp, intense, and persistent, reaching a peak typically in three to five minutes. The pain can be so sudden and intense that some people say that it's as if a bomb went off in their head. Cluster headache pain tends to affect only one side of the head with the typical attack lasting from a half hour to two hours. Stuffy nose, red eye, nausea, and tearing are often seen with cluster headaches. What often distinguishes a cluster headache from a migraine is the response to it: someone with a migraine tends to lie on a bed and remain still, whereas a cluster-attack sufferer often walks around the room. In the episodic form, there is a period of intense attacks that can last for two months. This is typically followed by a period of remission, or absence of attacks. In the chronic form, the attacks are more persistent without prolonged periods of remission. In about 70 percent of those affected, alcohol is identified as a precipitant. Additionally, many patients report that their attacks often happen at the same time each day. While many cluster attacks start during the day, about half occur at night, waking the victim up and disturbing his or her sleep.

Cluster headaches are believed to result from disorders of the hypothalamus and suprachiasmatic nucleus, structures found deep inside the brain. The rhythmic nature of cluster headache implicates these structures and the circadian rhythms they control. Circadian rhythms are controlled by our internal biological clock and influence many parts of our lives, such as sleep and blood pressure. Indeed, cluster headaches often occur during a particular time of day as well as season, suggesting a role for the biological clock in this disorder. Biological clock abnormalities are probably one reason why the "sleep" hormone melatonin can help cluster headaches, as several studies have found.

Hypothalamus
An ancient part of the brain located deep within the skull and primarily involved with temperature regulation.

From a chemical perspective, while multiple neurotransmitters are probably involved, as in migraines, disordered serotonin metabolism has been reported in cluster headaches. Finally, though cluster headaches are described as "vascular," investigations have not demonstrated any predictable blood-flow abnormalities in the disorder.

Therapy is aimed either at treating the acute attack or at preventing future attacks. Traditional medical therapy for acute cluster headache includes sumatriptan, prednisone, ergotamine, dihydroergotamine, verapamil, lithium, and inhaled oxygen. While many people do not consider inhaled oxygen a drug, most physicians would agree that oxygen is a medication. Multiple agents have also been used with variable success for the prevention of cluster headaches and include verapamil, lithium, steroids, and ergotamine agents. Natural therapies that have been reported to work for cluster headache include capsaicin and melatonin.

Cough-Related Headache

This type of headache is usually found in men and is related to head pain with sneezing, lifting, or coughing. Fortunately, these headaches only last seconds to minutes and then resolve. Though cough-related headache is typically a harmless problem, about 25 percent of individuals with cough headache may have a potentially serious brain disorder; hence, people with this syndrome should be evaluated by a physician.

Migraine Headache

Next to tension headache, migraine headaches are the most common type of headache and are experienced by 15 percent of women and 6 percent of men. Migraines are considered a "vascular" type of headache and are often chronic. While migraines are painful, they are generally benign and do not lead to more serious disease. The typical migraine has the following symptoms: photo-

Photophobia
Often seen in a migraine headache, a condition where light, especially bright light, exacerbates headache symptoms and disturbs the eyes.

phobia, pounding headache, visual changes, and nausea and vomiting (or both). A common feature of migraine headache is the "aura," which is a visual disturbance that precedes the headache. Rare migraine symptoms include diarrhea, confusion, seizures, and passing out.

The intensity of migraine pain ranges from mild to severe. Mild migraines are characterized by periodic throbbing but do not significantly impact quality of life. Conversely, severe migraines result in at least three headaches monthly, with severe pain that is accompanied by nausea and vomiting. Needless to say, severe migraines have a negative impact on the quality of life. Moderately severe migraines occupy a middle ground; such headaches range from moderate to severe, and are accompanied by nausea that can interfere with daily activities.

In rare instances, especially in familial hemiplegic migraine (FHM), migraine symptoms can mimic those of a stroke with weakness, numbness, or loss of vision. While these rare symptoms can occasionally last for days, they most commonly resolve in an hour. Genetics can be involved—the abnormality of FHM is localized to chromosome 19, which appears to be responsible for 50 percent of the cases. Indeed, multiple genetic defects have been described in migraine headache, and it appears that the syndrome results from a complex interplay between genes and the environment.

If you have migraines or know someone with migraines, chances are you realize that this disorder often runs in families. Indeed, migraine headaches have been inherited by many individuals, and the genetic basis of migraine headache is well documented in the scientific literature. In a typical pattern, a woman with a history of migraine headaches has a mother who has a similar history.

Many people have "nonclassic" migraine with complaints of a vice-like squeezing, similar to tension headaches. This is in part why some authorities consider migraine and tension headaches to be manifestations of the same disorder. While migraines can occur spontaneously, some people can identify triggers, such as red wine, sleep deprivation, and menstruation. Conversely, sleep, improved mood, and pregnancy have been reported to alleviate migraine headaches.

For decades it was believed that migraine headaches resulted from defects in the brain's blood flow. This is why migraines are still referred to as "vascular" headaches. It was proposed that both dilatation and constriction of the brain's blood flow were variously responsible for the syndrome we call "migraine headache." Adding credence to this theory are studies that demonstrate decreased blood flow in the brains of people who suffer from migraine. There are, however, people who suffer from migraine but have normal cerebral blood flow. While there are clearly blood flow abnormalities in migraine, whether or not these abnormalities are sufficient to produce migraine symptoms is hotly debated. What appears to be emerging from the literature today is that, although blood flow abnormalities are clearly present in migraine, they are only part of the picture.

A possible migraine mechanism is called the "neuronal theory of migraine." In this model, a wave of cerebral excitation is followed by a wave of inhibition. These waves are believed to originate deep in the brain stem and may be one of several processes operative in migraine headaches. Multiple other mechanisms, each of which enjoys a variable degree of support in the scientific literature, have also been implicated in migraines. These theories range from the roles of serotonin and dopamine to the activation of specific brain stem nuclei and the sympathetic nervous system. Some researchers suspect that, because of a genetic defect, many people who

suffer from migraines are unable to effectively regulate neurotransmitter concentrations; this con-
cept is known as the "empty
neuron theory."

Neurotransmitter
*Typically, a chemical
produced in the brain;
it is a chemical messen-
ger responsible for trans-
mitting signals between
cells of the central and
peripheral nervous
system.*

The role of serotonin in
migraine has been extensively studied, and abnormalities
in serotonin metabolism have
been clearly identified. Our
ability to understand the role
serotonin plays in migraine
has allowed pharmaceutical
researchers to develop triptan
drugs, which act on certain types of serotonin
receptors, thereby helping to relieve migraine
symptoms. This knowledge has also allowed alternative and complementary healthcare practition-
ers to use 5-HTP, a serotonin precursor, to treat
migraine and other headache disorders. Indeed,
serotonin-sensitive neural pathways have been
described throughout the brain and interact at
important locations. These serotonin-related con-
nections can in part explain many of the symptoms associated with migraine.

Another neurotransmitter that has received
considerable attention in migraine headaches is
dopamine. Both hypersensitivity to dopamine and
genetic abnormalities in dopa-
mine receptors have been described in individuals who suffer
from migraines. Stimulation of
dopamine can induce migrainelike symptoms. As a result of
these findings, drugs that coun-
teract or antagonize dopamine
action have been developed for
treating migraines.

Dopamine
*A neurotransmitter
that is linked to pain
and depression. Dys-
function in dopamine
metabolism has been
described in head-
ache syndromes.*

Although we are still working out the complex
mechanisms behind migraine headaches, emerging evidence has implicated a "hyperexcitable

brain" as being responsible for this painful syndrome. This hyperexcitable state probably results from imbalances between excitatory amino acid–mediated stimuli and inhibitory gamma-aminobutyric acid (GABA) stimuli. As in the research we've seen in cluster headaches, some experts blame derangements in the pineal gland for migraine headaches. Indeed, researchers have found low melatonin levels, the hormone secreted by the pineal gland, in people with migraine. Eventually, we will probably find that migraines result from a number of abnormalities, such as magnesium deficiency, nitric oxide derangements, and mitochondrial abnormalities.

Pineal Gland
A glandular structure, located deep in the brain, responsible for the secretion of melatonin.

Many people who suffer from migraines will tell you they have triggers that can set off an attack. Included in this list of triggers are hunger, low blood sugar, alcohol, stress, exercise, and sleep deprivation. Surprisingly, although a good night's sleep is known to help relieve migraine symptoms, too much sleep can trigger an attack. Other people, however, will experience migraines for no apparent reason.

Melatonin
Sometimes referred to as the "hormone of sleep"; it helps to regulate the biological clock.

As previously noted, foods are another notorious migraine trigger. Included in this list are foods that contain nitrates or MSG. Some people with migraine are also sensitive to chocolate and cheese, whereas others will tell you that smells or bright lights can trigger an attack. For some women, menstruation is a trigger for migraine, and is commonly known as a menstrual migraine. Finally, not only is your grandmother's bunion sensitive to weather changes, but her headaches may be as well, as some people with migraine are exceptionally sensitive to changes in barometric pressure.

Migraine headaches are broken down into several distinct subtypes. The most prevalent type is the "common migraine," otherwise known as "migraine *without* aura." In common migraine, there are no neurological findings prior to headache onset. The head pain is typically described on one side of the head and pulsating with mild to severe intensity. The pain is often made worse by motion and it is not uncommon to find the person involved lying motionless in a dark, quiet room. Another typical feature of common migraine is nausea, with or without vomiting. Sensitivity to light and sound may also be present, and are known as photophobia and phonophobia, respectively. Common migraine tends to be chronic with the average attack lasting four to seventy-two hours.

Another common type of migraine is the "classic migraine" or "migraine *with* aura." This type of headache is similar to the common migraine, except that prior to pain onset the patient will have neurological abnormalities known as an "aura." The aura can manifest as visual or motor changes or involve strange sensations. Of these, visual abnormalities are most common and typically involve blind spots (for example, scotoma) or hallucinations. The scotoma usually begins in the center of the vision field and gradually expands in size, often assuming a "C" shape. The edges of the blind spot may glow and change color as the scotoma begins to move and disappear. While other types of visual disturbances exist with auras, this scenario is typical and is called a "fortification spectrum." Scotomas usually last no more than thirty minutes, are harmless, and are believed to arise from nerves in the occipital lobe, the back part of the brain.

Other less common types of migraines include the basilar migraine and carotidynia. In basilar migraine, the patient will have symptoms, such as double vision, dizziness, confusion, ringing in the ears, or difficulty with speech. These symptoms can last up to thirty minutes, after which the headache occurs. Basilar migraine pain is often localized to the base of the skull. These symptoms can last several days but ultimately completely resolve. A rare form of basilar migraine is called a Bickerstaff migraine. This syndrome typically affects teenage girls and is accompanied by basilar migraine and blindness. Like the basilar migraine, full recovery is the rule.

Carotidynia, also known as a "facial migraine," is characterized by facial pain that is localized to the lower or upper jaw or neck. The pain of carotidynia varies from a dull throb to an "ice-pick" like quality. The attacks last from minutes to hours and may occur several times weekly. The syndrome may also be accompanied by pain over the carotid artery in the neck. This type of migraine is normally seen in people between the ages of forty and seventy.

The best way to treat a migraine is to remove the precipitant, if it is known. For instance, many people with migraine will say that stress is a common trigger. Reducing stress, a feat not so simple in a stressful world, is the answer to this problem. Nevertheless, multiple stress-relieving techniques exist, such as biofeedback. There are also a variety of traditional and alternative therapies that can help relieve migraine symptoms, such as magnesium and butterbur, which we will discuss later in this book.

Postconcussion Headache

This type of headache usually follows head trauma, such as can occur in a car accident. Indeed, following even a minor head injury, some people develop a syndrome of dizziness, headache, and memory dysfunction that can last from weeks to years after the injury. The name "postconcussion" is misleading, as this syndrome can occur even if consciousness is not lost as a result of the trauma. In the vast majority of cases, diagnostic studies such as CT and MRI are perfectly normal and the syndrome ultimately resolves on its own. A potentially serious disorder that can also cause a similar set of symptoms is a chronic subdural hematoma, which is a slowly growing collection of blood just under the skull. This is why following a head injury, close contact with a healthcare professional with diagnostic imaging is necessary. With the exception of subdural hematoma, the cause of postconcussion headache is not known.

Orgasm/Sex-Related Headache

Also known as a coital headache, this syndrome affects men four times more often than women. The typical sex-related headache occurs suddenly around the time of orgasm, lasts a few minutes, and then subsides. The bad news is that these headaches can interrupt your sex life. The good news is that orgasm-related headaches are almost always benign and not indicative of a serious disorder.

Tension Headache

There is little doubt that tension headaches are one of the most common types of headaches and are experienced by virtually every individual at some time. While females have more headaches than men, tension headaches can occur in any age group. The classic symptom of a tension headache is a tight, bandlike head pain. Tension headaches tend to be chronic; the pain occurs globally, on both sides of the head. It is not uncommon to hear people complain that their headache feels as if their head is in a vice. Like a migraine, tension headache pain is gradual in onset and can last from hours to days. Similarly, the pain can vary in intensity from a mild annoyance to severe head pain. Although a relationship between tension headache and anxiety or depression (or both) has been documented, most people with tension headache are not anxious or depressed.

As mentioned previously, controversy exists over the relationship between tension and migraine headache. Some investigators consider these headaches to be manifestations of a similar disorder. Other experts believe that tension and migraine headaches are distinct syndromes. While the exact cause of tension headaches is still not known, head and neck muscular abnormalities have been described.

As you will learn later, tension headache often responds best to relaxation techniques such as biofeedback and massage. Traditional therapies include acetaminophen, NSAIDs, muscle relaxants, and occasional antidepressants. Caffeine is another agent that has been used successfully for both tension and migraine headache. Multiple alternative therapies also exist for tension headache; peppermint oil and L-5-hydroxytryptophan have both demonstrated efficacy.

The Psychology of Headaches

Multiple studies have established that in some people, there is a definite relationship between depression and head pain. This is not to say that your symptoms are all in your head so to speak; however, in some people, emotions can play a role in their headaches. While emotions can affect head pain, we also know that chronic headaches can lead to mood swings, and even depression. In someone who suffers from depression and headaches, it is challenging to determine if the headache caused the depression or the depression caused the headache. It is perhaps most important that physicians and patients recognize the role psychological factors can play in headaches. Awareness of this role has led many experts to observe that antidepressant drugs are effective in treating migraine and tension headache. Similarly, the association between headaches and depression may have led to the use of natural supplements such as L-5-hydroxytryptophan to successfully treat tension and migraine headaches, as has been reported.

CHAPTER 3

NATURAL SUPPLEMENTS FOR HEADACHE RELIEF

Many people turn to natural remedies because they are not satisfied with traditional Western approaches, and it is not surprising that integrative medicine has exploded over the past three decades. I'm one of those triple A–personality New-York-City doctors raised by large, stodgy, academic medical centers that fed us a steady diet of traditional Western Medicine. If I didn't know that tobacco and alcohol were harmful, I'd probably resemble Winston Churchill—sitting in some dark, smoky, back room with a very large cigar in one hand and a glass of scotch in the other, growling with disdain at anything that even hinted of integrative medicine.

Today, I'm evidence that even old-school New-York-City boys can turn over a new leaf. When I started writing about integrative medicine six years ago, I was skeptical about vitamins, minerals, herbs, and any other therapy that didn't involve high technology or at least a powerful pharmaceutical with lots of juicy side effects. As I researched my articles, it slowly dawned on me that some of this stuff really works. I was pleasantly surprised to learn that the people who perform this research have backgrounds similar to mine and suffer the same trials and tribulations every scientist faces when seeking that elusive thing called truth. Needless to say, it has been a learning experience that forever changed the way I look at health and medicine. So, before we delve into the nitty-gritty of supplements and allergies, let us briefly examine the challenges scientists and physicians face when conducting such research.

Research Challenges

Vitamin and mineral deficiencies usually occur in one of three ways in humans: inadequate intake, improper absorption, or increased demand. Investigators have conducted research into vitamin and mineral supplements to determine if replacing a deficient agent can improve or eliminate headaches. One of the problems associated with supplement research is that if an individual is deficient in substance A, chances are they are also deficient in substance X, Y, and Z. In other words, vitamin and mineral deficiencies do not occur in a vacuum because the dietary or medical derangements that created the deficiency usually cause other deficiencies. Knowing this, you can see why it is difficult to study one particular deficiency without considering other deficiencies. When you have five or six different deficiencies, this mix rapidly complicates the research.

The second challenge facing supplement research is to take into account that proper neurologic function rests not on a single nutrient, but on an entire symphony of vitamins and minerals that are responsible for overall health. Consequently, it is very difficult to test the impact of supplementing a particular vitamin or mineral on headaches.

Further complicating the study of supplements, most studies report that a particular supplement benefited some but not all study participants. For example, in a study examining the effect of vitamin X on headaches, the authors may report that only 54 percent of the participants had a favorable response to supplements. This is a common finding, because the medical condition we call "headache" is the shared endpoint of multiple abnormal biological pathways. Many roads lead to headaches and every individual has his or her own unique set of genetic and environmental influences that result in the expression of some, but not all, of these pathways. These unique pathways are the reason why we have multiple types of headaches that often respond to different treatments. Although variety may be the spice of life, multiple pathways present a special challenge to researchers, since we are still in the process of understanding how they work and interact. Headaches clearly result from a complex interplay between genes and environment, and this is why we see a particular supplement work for some, but not for all, people. The good news is that as our knowledge grows, we are beginning to understand that, while many roads lead to headaches, they tend to end at the same place, and some of our most successful therapies target these common pathways.

Nutrient researches also have to contend with the varying diets of study subjects. The ideal supplement study would examine two groups of identical people with identical medical conditions, nutrient deficiencies, and diets, while comparing the effect of supplementation versus no supplementation. Although it is relatively easy to find people with similar medical conditions, it's difficult to control and fully monitor individual diets. What's nice about animal studies is that one can totally control an animal's diet. That means all gerbils get *x* amount of grams of the same food each and every day, with only one group receiving the supplement. Theoretically, you could lock two groups of people in a cage and feed them identical diets, but this is obviously not an option. The other tough part about diets and research studies is that people cheat—boy do they cheat! Scientists do have mathematical models that correct data for different diets; however, dietary aberrations will always remain a potential source of confusion and error.

So What Are You Going to Do?

As with any emerging field of medicine, controversy exists over the true effect supplements have on headaches. Nevertheless, despite the complexities of nutrient research, a substantial body of literature indicates that for many people with headaches there are some supplements that can help. Given the number of potential supplements, it's natural to wonder, *How do I choose the supplements that are right for me?* Nobody wants to be popping fifty pills a day, so let me help you figure this out.

As an old-school physician, I strongly recommended that every person with headaches, in addition to a healthy diet, regular exercise, and adequate sleep, routinely supplement their diet with one or two agents. I suggest you ask a knowledgeable healthcare professional to help you choose one or two standard supplements that are tailored to your individual needs. I am recommending two agents, because these supplements tend to work better when used in combination. If you can find a supplement that satisfactorily rids you of headaches by itself—wonderful. However, what some people will need to do is take two or more supplements to achieve effective relief, a situation that is especially common for people who suffer from severe headaches.

What I'd like you to do is start taking two standard supplements that will not only help your headaches but also protect you against the diseases you're personally at risk for. Chances are your headaches will improve after one to two months of taking these supplements. After two months, if your symptoms are still not where you would like them to be, I suggest you continue taking your two standard agents while experimenting with additional individual supplements to see which vitamin or mineral offers your headaches the most bang for your buck. Give each supplement a four-week trial while recording your symptoms in your headache diary. I also suggest that you get tested for vitamin and mineral deficiencies and, with the aid of a skilled healthcare professional, correct any deficiency found.

Please remember that nutritional supplements are only a small part of the headache picture. The purpose of this book is to eliminate or markedly improve your headaches. The foundation of good health does not rest with supplements alone; rather, a healthy life demands a clean environment, good nutrition, regular exercise, and adequate sleep. Supplements can help people with headaches; however, they are only one piece of the complex puzzle we call health. That said, let's investigate the supplements that can potentially help alleviate your symptoms and improve your life.

Magnesium for Migraine Headache

Magnesium is needed to make bone, proteins, and ATP. Magnesium is also needed to activate the B vitamins. Found in beans, grains, dairy products, fish, meat, nuts, and dark-green veggies, magnesium is used in the treatment of heart failure and irregular heart rhythms.

ATP
The basic energy unit used by cells; it is one of the final end-products of the food we ingest.

Low magnesium levels have been found in patients with migraine and cluster headaches but not in those with tension headaches. According to one group, "up to 50 percent of patients during an acute migraine attack have lower levels of ionized magnesium." While research clearly indicates that intravenous magnesium can help abort some headaches, research regarding oral magnesium supplements is mixed; some studies report positive results while others report negative results. For instance, one 1996 study from Austria reported no difference in the number of migraine attacks between those in the group receiving placebo and those in the group treated with magnesium. Conversely, a placebo-controlled, clinical trial found that magnesium supplements reduced head pain, headache frequency, and premenstrual complaints in a group of women with menstrual migraine. Another placebo-controlled, multicenter, randomized, controlled trial in 1996 by A. Peikert, et al., using oral magnesium in migraine sufferers, reported a 41.6 percent reduction in attack frequency compared to 15.8 percent for the placebo group. Medication use as well as the number of days with migraine also decreased. Likewise, the authors reported a reduction in "duration and intensity" of attacks, but the differences between the treated group and the placebo group were not statistically significant.

Despite these mixed findings, authors from the New York Headache Center wrote, "because of the excellent safety profile and low cost and despite the lack of definitive studies, we feel that a trial of oral magnesium supplementation can be recommended in the majority of migraine sufferers." Given the strong association with magnesium deficiency and headache, anyone with chronic headaches should consider having their magnesium level checked. While no trials on magnesium for cluster headache have been reported, given the correlation between low magnesium and cluster headache, a trial is warranted.

The relationship between tension headache and magnesium is still being investigated. Some authors believe that derangements in magnesium metabolism play a role in tension headache, and that such derangements can be corrected through supplementation; however, clinical trials establishing this benefit are lacking.

Dosage

Most authorities suggest supplementing with 250–

350 milligrams of magnesium daily. Since vitamin B$_6$ (pyridoxine) aids in magnesium absorption, take 10–25 milligrams of pyridoxine with magnesium. A daily multivitamin/mineral supplement is also recommended, since magnesium competes with other minerals like calcium for absorption and you want to be sure of obtaining the other vitamins and minerals you need. The most common side effect of magnesium is diarrhea. Rare side effects include burping, depression, excess gas, lethargy, nausea, stomach cramps, vomiting, and weakness. If you have kidney problems, talk to your doctor before taking magnesium. Do not take magnesium supplements if you are having diarrhea or have a history of high-magnesium blood levels.

Vitamin B$_2$ (Riboflavin) for Migraine Headache

Besides being needed for amino acid metabolism, riboflavin helps convert sugar into ATP. Used to treat anemia, it is suspected that riboflavin "improves neuronal energy production," thereby helping to prevent migraines. Two studies exist regarding this vitamin and migraine headache. The first study was published in 1998 in the journal *Neurology*. This was a randomized, controlled clinical trial conducted in Belgium. In this study, forty-nine patients were treated with riboflavin for three months after which 68.2 percent reported positive "global improvement." The second study was a placebo-controlled, randomized, clinical trial in fifty-five people with migraine. Not only did riboflavin supplements reduce migraine attack frequency but the number of headache days was reduced in 59 percent of the vitamin group compared to only 15 percent for placebo group. Two participants had minor side effects consisting of diarrhea and excess urination. It is suspected that riboflavin works by increasing mitochondrial energy function. Mitochondria are known as the cell "powerhouse" and mitochondrial dysfunction is suggested as one of several mechanisms behind migraine attacks. The authors concluded that "because of its high efficacy, excellent tolerability, and low cost, riboflavin is an interesting option for migraine prophylaxis."

Dosage

The typical dosage of riboflavin in these studies was 400 milligrams daily. Side effects are rare and vitamin B_2 is usually taken as part of a B complex vitamin.

Vitamin B_{12} (Cyanocobalamin) for Migraine Headache

If you've got nerve, you need B_{12}, a vital vitamin for normal nerve function. Besides making sure you've got nerve, vitamin B_{12} also helps ensure you have a functioning heart, working with vitamin B_6 and folic acid to reduce homocysteine, an amino acid that can increase your risk of heart disease. Cyanocobalamin deficiency is associated with fatigue—some people use B_{12} injections to treat chronic fatigue. Commonly found in meat, fish, and dairy products, vitamin B_{12} has also been used for depression and pernicious anemia.

With the exception of several studies in the 1950s and 1960s, the only modern study on vitamin B_{12} for headache was published in 2002. This study by P. van der Kuy, et al., in the Netherlands, investigated twenty patients who had migraines two to eight times monthly and who were treated with an intranasal solution of B_{12} for three months. During this period, 53 percent of the patients had a 50 percent or more reduction in attack frequency. The authors also noted reduced medication use, attack duration, and number of days with headache. These scientists suspect that B_{12} is effective at preventing migraines because it is a nitrous oxide scavenger. Although this is the first pilot study, it is encouraging news for vitamin B_{12} and migraine sufferers.

Dosage

Recommendations for B_{12} supplementation vary, depending on the condition treated. Strict vegetarians usually require 2–3 micrograms a day, whereas for people with pernicious anemia a dosage of 1,000 micrograms daily is standard. Some authorities recommend that the elderly take 10–25 micrograms of B_{12} daily. Side effects are rare with oral B_{12}; however, diarrhea and occasional allergic reactions to injections occur. Do not take vitamin B_{12} if you are allergic to cobalt.

Vitamin D and Calcium for Migraine Headache

Of all the body's minerals, calcium is the most abundant, and almost all our calcium resides in our bones. Besides being vital for healthy bones and teeth, calcium plays a pivotal role in muscle contraction, nerve conduction, and blood clotting. Used to treat celiac disease, osteoporosis, and rickets, there is also emerging evidence that calcium-rich diets may protect against colon polyps. Most of our dietary calcium comes from dairy products; however, sardines, tofu, and leafy green vegetables represent additional sources. Vitamin D is the calcium gatekeeper, ensuring a healthy balance of calcium between the blood and bone. For people with headaches, there are two case reports of a calcium and vitamin D combination being used to treat migraines.

The first report, which was published in the journal *Headache*, involved two women with menstrual migraines. According to the author, after treatment with calcium and vitamin D, both women had a "major reduction in their headache attacks as well as premenstrual symptomatology."

The second report was also published in *Headache* and involved two women who had "excruciating migraine headaches," which were treated with calcium and vitamin D. According to the researchers, these women experienced a "dramatic reduction in migraine frequency and duration."

Dosage

The typical vitamin D dosage is 200–1,000 IU daily. Side effects include constipation, dry mouth, headaches, vomiting, and weight loss. If you have a history of heart disease, hyperparathyroidism, kidney disease, sarcoidosis, or intend to take more than 1,000 IU a day, talk to your doctor before using vitamin D. Do not take vitamin D if you have kidney failure or a history of elevated blood calcium or phosphate levels.

Of all the calcium supplements on the market, calcium citrate and calcium citrate/malate appear to have the best absorption, Most people take 800–1,000 milligrams of calcium daily when supplementing. The most common calcium-related side effects are bloating, constipation, and gas.

Since vitamin D is necessary for calcium absorption, 400 IU of vitamin D is usually taken with calcium. A daily multivitamin/mineral supplement is also recommended, since calcium competes with other minerals for absorption.

Niacin for Migraine Headache

Found naturally in brewer's yeast, fish, meat, and peanuts, niacin is used to treat alcohol withdrawal and high cholesterol. Although the literature regarding niacin and migraine is limited, it has been encouraging. In 2003 the Mayo Clinic published a case report of a patient "whose migraine headache responded dramatically to sustained-release niacin as preventative treatment." It is suspected that niacin helps increase plasma serotonin, low levels of which have been described in migraine sufferers. In 2001, another study followed, by A. Gedye, which used a combination of tryptophan, niacin, calcium, caffeine, and acetylsalicylic acid (aspirin) to treat twelve people with migraine. According to the report, 75 percent of those treated "had significant benefit." Despite these intriguing findings, the jury is still out on niacin and further research is clearly needed. I have no objection to people with migraines taking niacin: if it doesn't help your headaches, it's bound to drop your cholesterol level.

Dosage

Most people start with 100 milligrams of niacin, once daily, and gradually increase the dose to 100–300 milligrams three times a day. Make sure you take niacin with meals and at least two glasses of water. Do not take more than 1,000 milligrams a day without consulting a physician. A newer type of niacin called inositol hexaniacinate appears to offer the same health benefits without the side effects associated with niacin.

The most notorious side effect of niacin is flushing; however, headache, stomach pain, and vomiting can also occur with dosages as low as 50 milligrams a day. Additional rare side effects can occur with higher dosages and include diabetes, diarrhea, dry skin, eye problems, gout, headache, irregular heart rhythms, liver toxicity, low blood pressure, muscle injury, nausea, skin rash, stomach pain/ulcers, and vomiting. Alcohol and hot drinks often increase flushing, whereas 125–350 milligrams of aspirin taken twenty to thirty minutes prior to niacin may prevent flushing.

Have your physician periodically check your liver function and evaluate side effects while taking niacin. Do not use niacin if you have bleeding problems, liver disease, low blood pressure, or stomach ulcers. Finally, talk to your doctor prior to taking niacin if you have diabetes, gallbladder disease, gout, jaundice, liver problems, heart disease, tartrazine sensitivity, or a history of stomach ulcers or bleeding.

About Herbal Headache Remedies

Many of the drugs we use to treat medical illness literally have their roots in herbs found in the plant kingdom, and these herbs contain molecules that, when purified or synthesized, we call a drug. Given this consideration, it is important to treat herbs with the same respect and caution as we do our most potent pharmaceuticals. Prior to the era of pharmaceuticals civilization, through millions of years of trial and error, people have discovered that certain plants have medicinal properties. Only through the emergence of modern chemistry have we been able to isolate and synthesize the magic our ancestors discovered. As technology advanced, not only did we discover the active ingredients behind these medicinal herbs but we were also able to isolate, synthesize, and ultimately manipulate these agents, often enhancing their therapeutic benefit and eliminating side effects.

Synthesis, however, can result in toxic waste products that are harmful to the environment. Conversely, synthesis has dramatically reduced the economic and environmental costs of some drugs. Nevertheless, there are, and probably will always be, problems with the way we make and market pharmaceutics. Although the pharmaceutical industry isn't perfect, certainly, if it were not for modern drugs, many of the people who are walking this Earth would not be here today. Stop and think for a moment about all the people who would have died were it not for antibiotics, cancer drugs, or heart medications.

The same can be said of the herbal industry. Integrative therapies and their associated products represent a multibillion dollar industry that rivals the pharmaceutical industry. Like pharmaceutical companies, the herbal industry has its strengths and weaknesses. Medicinal herbs frequently offer consumers products that are often not available elsewhere. Medicinal herbs are also usually preservative and additive free, an important consideration for people with headaches.

Problems exist, however. One of the greatest challenges faced by the herbal industry is that of standardization, and a consumer can never be certain how much active ingredient they are getting from some preparations. For pharmaceuticals, however, strict formulary standards exist. The downside to modern pharmaceuticals is that they often contain preservatives and food colorings that can spell trouble for people with allergies, a problem less commonly found in "natural" products. While the vast majority of manufacturers are responsible, there are occasional disturbing reports of adulterated and mislabeled herbal products finding their way to market.

As for efficacy, we are fortunately beginning to see serious, rigorous studies on herbal products published in respected journals like the *Journal of the American Medical Association*. Although these reports are encouraging, herbal research is still in its infancy and documenting efficacy often takes years of research and controversy to achieve.

Finally, the extraction of herbs for direct use and for the development and production of medications by pharmaceutical companies can have a devastating impact on the environment. For example, the herb goldenseal (*Hydrastis canadensis*) is becoming endangered because of the extent to which it has been sought out for its medicinal properties. Again, there are two sides to every story. Granted, the herbal industry is far from perfect; however, if it were not for botanicals many of the people who are walking this Earth would not be here today. Stop and think for a moment about all the lives herbs have saved through the millennia.

This is the balanced approach to integrative and traditional medicine that I hope to share with you. As we walk through alternative and traditional therapies, I want your eyes wide open with an appreciation of their strengths and weaknesses. Like vitamins, minerals, and pharmaceuticals, the herb that works for your friend may not work for you. Despite their potential shortcomings, you are about to learn that herbs can help people with headaches. If you decide to take the herbal route, I suggest you do so under the guidance of a healthcare professional who is familiar with herbal therapy. Remember, the line between herb and drug is often blurred and many of our most powerful drugs had a humble start as a "weed" in somebody's backyard.

Butterbur (*Petasites hybridus*) for Migraine Headache

Butterbar is a shrub found in Asia, Europe, and North America that was used in the Middle Ages to treat plague. Fortunately, plague is rare, and today butterbur has found a role in the treatment of migraine headaches, asthma, and bowel disorders. Of particular interest, the leaves of this shrub can attain a diameter of three feet, and the term "butterbur" derives from the use of these leaves to wrap butter in the days before refrigeration.

It is believed that the medicinal qualities of butterbur reside in the petasines, agents that inhibit leukotriene synthesis and have anti-inflammatory action. Besides relieving pain, this herb has been used as an antispasmodic in urological and gastrointestinal disorders. As for headaches, one trial by W. Grossman et al., reported positive results for butterbur in

Leukotrienes *Substances produced by the body that are involved in inflammatory reactions.*

migraine. This placebo-controlled, randomized, double-blind, clinical study examined sixty patients who were given a *Petasites hybridus* extract twice daily for twelve weeks. According to the authors, migraine-attack frequency decreased by as much as 60 percent. These researchers also reported that butterbur was well tolerated, with "no adverse events." Although the results of this one study are encouraging, more studies are needed before we will know if butterbur will ever play a significant role in headache treatment.

Dosage

There have been rare reports of liver damage from this herb, so people with liver disease should avoid it. Most standardized extracts contain at least 7.5 milligrams of petasin and isopetasin; most authorities recommend taking 50–100 milligrams twice a day with meals. Do not use any preparation that contains pyrrolizidine alkaloids. Liver toxicity is the most important side effect and is caused by pyrrolizidine alkaloids, so they are normally removed from extracts. There are also reports of possible inhibition of testosterone synthesis, but these findings have not been confirmed in humans.

Capsaicin for Cluster and Migraine Headaches

It may surprise you to learn that something so hot and irritating as capsaicin has been successfully used in the prevention of cluster headache. This substance, which is found in red peppers, has been used for centuries to help relieve pain. It is suspected that topical application of capsaicin works its magic by depletion of substance P from sensory nerves, making the nerves insensitive to further stimulation. Because of its usefulness in treating

Substance P
A chemical that plays a leading role in pain sensation.

pain, capsaicin has been used to treat a variety of conditions including osteoarthritis, diabetic neuropathy, and postherpetic neuralgia.

Several studies have reported favorable results using intranasal capsaicin solutions for cluster headache. One multicenter, double-blind, randomized study from the Michigan Pain and Neurological Institute examined the effect of intranasal capsaicin in twenty-eight people with cluster headaches. These researchers found that the treatment group had a 55.5 percent reduction in the number of cluster headaches by day seven of treatment. Their results become even more impressive over time, reaching a 70.6 percent reduction by day twenty. According to the report, the most common side effects were tearing and nasal burning. Another study, published in 1993 from the Massachusetts General Hospital, found that intranasal capsaicin resulted in "significantly less severe" cluster headaches after eight to fifteen days of use. In this study, intranasal capsaicin was most effective when used episodically as opposed to chronically.

Another randomized, multicenter, double-blind, controlled trial, by S. Diamond, et al., tested intranasal capsaicin for treatment of acute migraine. This study examined thirty-four people with migraine headache and found that, after two hours, 55.6 percent had "decreased pain severity," with 22.2 percent of the subjects being "pain free." The results were even more impressive four hours after dosing, with 72.7 percent of the patients having less pain and 33.0 percent being pain free. Although no major side effects were observed, 91.2 percent of the subjects had nasal burning, and 44.1 percent reporting tearing. Although these researchers found that intranasal capsaicin was effective in treating acute migraine, they also wrote that given its mechanism of action, intranasal capsaicin "should be substantially more effective for prophylaxis than acute treatment of migraine."

Dosage

To use intranasal capsaicin, you may need to tolerate some combination of burning, sneezing, and nasal secretions at first, but these side effects often go away after several days. Most studies have administered intranasal capsaicin daily, as needed. Speak with a knowledgeable healthcare practitioner if you're interested in this therapy.

Feverfew (*Tanacetum parthenium*) for Migraine Headache

Related to sunflower, feverfew has been used as a medicinal herb for centuries. Despite this long history, the literature regarding feverfew for headaches has shown mixed results. For instance, one randomized, placebo-controlled, double-blind trial, published in the prestigious journal *The Lancet*, examined the impact of feverfew on migraine headache frequency in fifty-nine individuals who took supplements for four months. Supplementation reduced the number and severity of attacks; however, attack duration and vomiting were unchanged. No serious side effects with feverfew were noted during this study. Another study, by V. Pfaffenrath, et al., found that feverfew was only effective in patients who had four or more migraines monthly. These findings led the authors to conclude that feverfew "failed to show a significant migraine prophylactic effect."

An extensive analysis of the literature by the highly regarded Cochrane Database concluded that "the efficacy of feverfew for the prevention of migraine has not been established beyond reasonable doubt." Conversely, another major review of the literature concluded that "feverfew is likely to be effective in the prevention of migraine." Given the conflicting reports in the literature, one

can only say that for people with migraine headaches, a trial of feverfew may be worthwhile. The
herb has a low side-effect profile; nausea and
stomach upset are the most common ones. You
should not take feverfew if you are on blood thinners, such as warfarin, aspirin, or NSAIDs.

Dosage

Dosage varies according to the preparation; however, the typical dosage for feverfew leaves is 350
milligrams daily.

Peppermint Oil for Tension Headache

Peppermint is a hybrid of spearmint and water
mint that was first grown in England during the
1700s. Because peppermint is theorized to have
muscle-relaxant activity, several researchers de-
cided to investigate it for possible treatment of
tension headaches. One randomized, controlled,
clinical trial by H. Gobel, et al., in 1996, examined

Use of Placebos in Clinical Studies

An inert or inactive substance, often given during a clinical trial. It is used to distinguish a true
response to a drug or supplement versus the
effect that results from simple chance. In many
studies, the group is divided between placebo
and treatment group. One group is given the
placebo whereas the other is given the treatment agent. These groups are then followed for
a certain period of time after which they are
examined for a particular outcome and the differences between the group who received the
placebo versus those who received the treatment are compared. (Of course, study designs
can be much more complicated than this; however, this simple explanation is applicable to
most studies.)

---

a peppermint and eucalyptus oil topical preparation in thirty-two individuals. Although the combination did not have a significant impact on pain sensitivity, the authors noted that the mixture had a "muscle-relaxing and mentally relaxing effect." This same study noted that, when using a topical ethanol and peppermint oil combination, "a significant analgesic effect with a reduction in sensitivity to headache" resulted.

More encouraging results were reported by a German group in another randomized, placebo-controlled clinical trial in forty-one people with tension headache. According to the study, topical peppermint oil with ethanol "significantly reduced clinical headache intensity . . . after 15 minutes." Equally impressive, "there was no significant difference between the efficacy of 1,000 milligrams of acetaminophen and 10 percent peppermint oil in ethanol solution." The authors also wrote that the peppermint oil/ethanol solution was well tolerated, and ultimately, an effective treatment for tension headache.

Dosage

Usage varies according to the preparation; however, a typical regimen is to apply peppermint oil to the affected area up to four times daily.

L-5-Hydroxytryptophan (L-5-HTP; 5-HTP) for Migraine and Tension Headaches

5-HTP is used by the body to make serotonin—a brain chemical that plays an important role in mood, sleep, pain, and sexual behavior. Serotonin inhibits migraine-related pain pathways and is reported to help prevent several pain-related syndromes. Because of its pivotal role in pain transmission, 5-HTP has been studied for its ability to alleviate and prevent headache. One randomized, controlled trial in 124 individuals reported a significant improvement in intensity and duration of migraine in 71 percent of patients treated with 5-HTP. According to the authors, "these results suggest that 5-HTP could be a treatment of choice in the prophylaxis of migraine." A German trial by G. De Benedittis found that 5-HTP "resulted in a statistically significant reduction in frequency of migraine attacks." Finally, one group examined the efficacy of 5-HTP in people with migraine, mixed headache, psychogenic headache, and muscle-contraction headache. After two months of treatment, 48 percent of the individuals had 50 percent or greater reductions in headache symptoms.

In 2000, a report on chronic tension headache from the Portuguese Head Society stated that 5-HTP resulted in a "significant decrease in the consumption of analgesics." Likewise, this same study found a "significant decrease in the number of days with headache" for two weeks following 5-HTP treatment.

Dosage

Most people take 400–600 milligrams of 5-HTP daily for headache. As it is well absorbed in the gut, you can take this supplement with food. Side effects are uncommon, mild, and transient and mostly consist of anxiety, nausea, and insomnia. Do not take 5-HTP if you have liver or autoimmune disease. People who are taking antidepressants or serotonin-related agents should not take 5-HTP. Likewise, if you are pregnant or breast-feeding, this supplement should be avoided.

Coenzyme Q_{10} (CoQ_{10}) for Migraine Headache

Oxidant stress has been implicated in a wide variety of diseases including heart disease, aging, and cancer. Coenzyme Q_{10} is a powerful antioxidant, and there are numerous studies documenting its efficacy in managing high cholesterol, heart disease, and neurological disorders like Parkinson's disease. So far, there has been only one study regarding CoQ_{10} and headache. This clinical trial was done at Thomas Jefferson University in Philadelphia in 2002 and involved thirty-two patients with migraine who were supplemented with 150 milligrams of CoQ_{10} daily.

After three months of therapy, the average number of days with headache dropped from 7.34 to 2.95 days. Likewise, 61.3 percent of the participants had a 50 percent or greater reduction in number of days with migraine. The mean reduction in headache frequency was 13.1 percent by month one, jumping to 55.3 percent by month three, indicating that the longer CoQ_{10} was taken the more effective it became. No side effects were observed and the authors concluded that "coenzyme Q_{10} appears to be a good migraine preventive." Although additional human studies will be needed to further document the role of CoQ_{10} as a headache abolisher, the results from this respected institution are encouraging.

Dosage

The most common dose of coenzyme Q_{10} is 50–200 milligrams daily.

Omega-3 and Omega-6 Fatty Acids for Migraine Headache

Not all fats are created equal. Polyunsaturated fatty acids like omega-3 and omega-6 are what we call "good" fats, whereas saturated fats that are commonly found in baked goods like doughnuts and potato chips are "bad" fats. The best thing about fish is that it is rich in omega-3-fatty acids, a fat that may help you live longer. Just to give you a taste of what fish can do, one Harvard study examined the dietary habits 84,688 adults and found that people who ate fish two to four times a week slashed their risk of heart disease by 31 percent. That's something to shake your salmon at!

Considering the important role fish oils play in preserving overall health, eating fish is a win-win situation. Fish work their magic through essential fatty acids (EFAs) like omega-3 and omega-6. The chief omega-3 acids are eicosapentaenoic acid (EPA) and docosahexaenoic acid (DHA), and they can be found in anchovies, albacore tuna, herring, sardines, and salmon. You can even find omega-3 in flaxseed oil, walnut oil, and game meat. If you really want to suck down some heavy DHA and EPA, try the old favorite cod liver oil. While omega-6 is a good fat, too much omega-6 may increase your risk of heart disease and high blood pressure. Nevertheless, I strongly recommend that you maintain a healthy balance between the two omegas since these fats are essential.

Many theories exist as to why people get headaches. Although there are many more questions than answers, we do know that cytokines like leukotrienes are involved in some headaches. Some experts believe that cytokines are behind food-associated headaches. The good news is that besides protecting your heart, the oils found in fish can block leukotriene synthesis. This blocking process may be one of the mechanisms behind the findings in one randomized, controlled, clinical study, reported in 2002, that examined two months of fish-oil supplementation in twenty-three adolescents with migraine. These teenagers reported significant reductions in both headache frequency and intensity. Indeed, 87 percent had fewer headaches, 74 percent had reduced headache duration, and 83 percent had less severe headaches. Similar results were reported by these researchers for two months of olive oil use; 78 percent reported reduced frequency, 70 percent reported headache reduction, and 65 percent reported reduced severity.

Cytokines
Substances released by immune-system cells that are involved in inflammation.

Dosage

For supplementation, most authorities recommend approximately 10 grams of fish oil daily. Some experts go a little higher, suggesting 2–9 grams of omega-3 and 9–18 grams of omega-6. You can meet these requirements simply by mixing a tablespoon of flaxseed oil with your favorite food daily. Nutritional experts also recommend washing your fish oil down with an antioxidant such as vitamin E to preserve the potency of the oils, which are extremely sensitive to oxygen degradation. If taking a pill is not for you, remember that oily fish like salmon and cod are rich in essential fatty acids.

Melatonin for Migraine, Tension, and Cluster Headaches

Melatonin is the hormone of sleep that is secreted by the pineal gland, which is located deep within the brain. Melatonin has long been used to treat sleep-related disorders, and evidence is emerging that melatonin can help people with migraine and tension headaches. Disturbances in the natural secretion of melatonin are reported in migraine, and some authorities suspect that pineal dysfunction may play a role. Likewise, low melatonin levels have been described in people with migraines and cluster headaches.

A 1998 study from the Netherlands reported that melatonin supplements helped relieve headache symptoms in thirty patients with sleep disorders. According to the report, three women in this group who had chronic tension headache found that their symptoms "disappeared" after two weeks of supplementation. Likewise, a male patient, who had twice-weekly migraines, reported only three migraines for a twelve-month period. Another patient reported reduced cluster headache duration during the trial. Despite this finding, reports are mixed regarding melatonin and cluster headache. For instance, a 2002 placebo-controlled clinical trial in nine people with cluster headache failed to show any benefit from melatonin. Conversely, one review article from the Mayo Clinic reported that melatonin "may be useful" in cluster headache. One small trial from Thomas Jefferson Medical Center, my alma mater, reported that two patients who suffered from cluster headache had their symptoms "alleviated" with melatonin. Another double-blind, placebo-controlled study in twenty patients with cluster headache reported a significant reduction in headache frequency, with a trend toward decreased medication use. Fifty percent of those treated with melatonin had a decline in attack frequency after three to five days with "no further attacks until melatonin was discontinued." According to the report, no side effects were reported.

The mechanisms behind melatonin's success are complicated; however, it is suspected that pain receptor changes as well as shifts in the biological clock play a role. Few side effects are reported with melatonin, the most common being lethargy. The association between melatonin and reduced sex drive, abdominal pain, and headache are less clear.

Dosage

Most people take 3 milligrams of melatonin prior to going to bed. Do not take melatonin if you have diabetes or glucose intolerance.

SAMe (S-Adenosylmethionine) for Migraine Headache

SAMe plays a pivotal role in many biochemical pathways and is involved in the manufacture of dopamine. As you may recall, dopamine dysfunction is described in headache and plays a crucial role in depression. SAMe is reported to increase dopamine levels, and this is believed to be one reason why this agent has been successfully used to treat depression, fibromyalgia, and arthritis.

There has only been one trial investigating SAMe in migraine. This 1986 trial by G. Gatto, et al., examined long-term supplementation and reported that SAMe "relieves pain in migraine sufferers . . . [but that] the benefits arise gradually and long-term treatment is required for therapeutic effectiveness." The authors speculate that SAMe works by modulation of 5-hydroxytryptamine, another agent known to have a beneficial effect in tension and migraine headaches.

Dosage

The typical SAMe dosage for migraine is 800 milligrams daily. Side effects are uncommon; the most frequent is stomach upset.

CHAPTER 4

Complementary, Alternative, and Traditional Headache Therapies

Behavioral therapy represents one of the great achievements in modern headache therapy, and offers results similar to those seen with traditional pharmacotherapy. On average, behavioral therapy results in a 35 to 50 percent reduction in migraine and tension headache. Its primary techniques are biofeedback, relaxation, and stress management. Multiple studies have demonstrated that the addition of behavioral therapy to drug therapy is synergistic with respect to relieving headache. Without a doubt, one of the most common triggers for headache, especially migraine, is stress. While it may not always be possible to remove stress from your life, there are several techniques that can not only help you relieve stress but also prevent headaches. These stress-relieving therapies hail from a variety of disciplines and include practices, such as biofeedback, massage therapy, and aerobic exercise.

> **Synergistic Action**
> *The total effect achieved by the methods used is greater than would be expected from simply adding their respective contributions together.*

Aerobic Exercise for General Health

Why exercise? Exercise is important not only to improve your headaches, as you will learn a little later, but also to protect you from this nation's number-one killer: heart disease. Regular exercise, especially aerobic exercise, strengthens your heart and lungs, adding healthy active years to your life.

Besides lowering your cholesterol and protecting you from heart disease, a healthy diet coupled with regular exercise will reduce your risk for cancer, diabetes, hypertension, and a whole host of other nasty ills. Exercise helps you sleep better, increases energy levels, and boosts your immune system. Exercise will make you look better naked and improve your sex life; now we're talking! If you have diabetes, hypertension, depression, fibromyalgia, or virtually any other chronic medical problem, exercise will make your condition more manageable. Even more important, exercise will make you feel good about yourself.

As soon as you start to exercise, as soon as you start to eat right, as soon as you make a commitment to healthy living, something magical happens: you take control of your life. By living healthy you say to the world, "I am the master of my fate. I have control—this is my responsibility." We need this attitude both to beat headaches and to be successful in everything we do.

There are three basic exercises that everyone should do regularly: aerobic exercise (such as running), anaerobic exercise (such as weight lifting), and stretching. Stretching is the orphan of exercise but is especially important and may help prevent injury. While all three exercises are important, if I were stuck on a desert island and could only do one exercise, it would be aerobic exercise. Aerobic exercises, such as walking, swimming, biking, and running, train your heart and lungs to work as a team. It's the aerobic exercise that will not only help your headaches but also add healthy active years to your life.

The type of aerobic exercise you choose depends on your level of physical fitness and personality. If you've been a dedicated couch potato for many years, I suggest you start by walking a half hour every day. You can walk in your neighborhood, in the mall, or in the woods. Where you choose to walk depends on where you live and how comfortable you are with walking. If you're in good shape and otherwise healthy, you can walk almost anywhere you please. If you have several medical conditions and haven't walked by yourself for some time, I suggest you walk where other people are present. After two weeks of daily walking, increase your walk to an hour every day. As the weeks pass, you'll want to increase the pace of your walk and throw in some hills for good measure. To make sure you're getting a good workout, you want to be breathing a little harder and faster than normal but not running out of breath and having to stop and rest.

Remember to stay well hydrated during exercise. Water is essential to life and if you're exercising correctly, you will probably work up a small sweat. Replacing water lost during exercise is especially important for asthmatics, not only to avoid heat exhaustion but also to prevent dehydration. The best replacement fluid is good old-fashioned water. Believe it or not, those fancy and expensive "sport" drinks can actually promote dehydration by shifting water from your body to the stomach in order to digest a whole bunch of sweeteners and electrolytes. Salt and electrolyte replacement is usually only needed by heavily perspiring athletes.

That said, back to aerobic exercise. After a couple months of dedicated walking, try biking, swimming, or joining an aerobics class. Once again, the type of activity you choose depends on your fitness level, personality, and where you live. If you live in a major city, biking may not be a realistic option and perhaps you'd be better off joining an aerobics class or joining a gym where you can swim. The nice thing about aerobics is that the classes come in all shapes and sizes, and you should have no problem finding an aerobics class that is right for you. Since swimming, biking, and aerobics tend to be more intense than walking, you won't have to do them as often to stay in shape—thirty to forty-five minutes every other day should be enough.

As with any type of exercise, your mantra should be "go slow and work your way up." For moderate-level aerobic exercise, you want to be breathing a little faster than you would be while walking. Don't be embarrassed to rest if you need to, it's better at first to develop aerobic strength rather than to pound your body into submission. My aversion to counting calories spills over into calculating heart rates. The fancy formulas for calculating target aerobic heart rate are unnecessary for most people. When exercising, I pay attention to what my body tells me. You know you're getting a good workout if you're breathing fast but can still carry a conversation. In other words, you want to feel like you're working but not like you're dying. If you can't catch your breath or complete a sentence, you're exercising too hard and need to slow down. Unless you're in excellent competitive-level shape, leave this heart-pounding, body-bashing stuff to the athletes. For the average person who wants to stay fit and does not intend to engage in high-intensity sports, I recommend sticking to moderate-level aerobic exercise. Moderate-level aerobic exercise offers similar health benefits to high-intensity aerobic exercise without the risk of injury.

Before you start attacking the Stairmaster, let's make sure you've been performing mid- to high-level aerobic exercise with some weight training and stretching thrown in for good measure. In other words, don't just roll out of bed one morning and decide that after ten years of sitting in front of the tube you're going to run marathons. This is a good way to get hurt; you really risk your life if you go from couch potato to superman overnight.

If you've been exercising regularly for the past year, and you have no other medical problems that would stop you from exercising, then there's no reason why you can't push yourself to the next level. Of course, it's always a good idea to talk to your doctor before embarking on an exercise program, especially one where you intend to push your body hard.

Which exercises you choose depends on your personality and availability. With aerobic exercise I like to mix things up and try not to do the same exercise every day. When you perform the same exercise daily, your body adapts and you don't get an efficient workout. Different exercises keep your body on its toes, forcing it to constantly change. Run one day, pound the Stairmaster the next, rest one day, then bike the next day—mix it up! Cross training is good for you!

If you're serious about exercise, I strongly recommend joining a gym. Quality exercise equipment can be pricey, and the machinery needed to perform multiple exercises can be found in most gyms. There's also a safety issue. If something "bad" happens, it's probably going to happen the first few days that you start to hammer yourself, and it's preferable to have other people around rather than being home alone.

Gyms can also be useful during air-quality alert days when it may be dangerous to exercise outdoors. And an extra plus for gyms: it's nice to interact with like-minded individuals, supporting each other and learning from each other's successes and mistakes. In fact, you might think about initially hiring a personal trainer to teach you how to exercise safely and correctly.

Aerobic Exercise for Migraine and General Headaches

Now for the nitty-gritty on exercise and headache: Multiple studies have documented the beneficial effects of aerobic exercise for migraine. One trial examined one hour of aerobic exercise three times weekly in migraine sufferers. Accordingly, "intensity, frequency, and duration of pain" was reduced significantly. In this study, the authors suspected that increased nitrous oxide levels were responsible for improved symptoms. Another potential benefit of aerobic exercise is that it may alter mitochondrial function. Mitochondrial dysfunction is reported in migraine patients and may be related to symptom severity. An additional benefit of aerobic exercise is that it can help relieve fatigue. Fatigue is a common problem seen in more than 85 percent of migraine patients.

Mitochondria
Energy-producing "factories" located in the body's cells.

Without a doubt, the best treatment for migraine, and for any medical condition, is a multidisciplinary approach. Such an approach is the philosophy of a group of researchers from Canada who studied a program of exercise, stress management, relaxation therapy, diet, and massage therapy in forty-one patients with migraine. According to their report, these patients experienced statistically significant positive changes in "pain frequency, pain intensity, pain duration, functional status, quality of life, health status, pain related disability, and depression"—changes that persisted during the three-month follow-up period.

Finally, one major review published in the *Medical Clinics of North America* reported that "there is little doubt, however, that aerobic exercise offers effective relief for many stress-provoked conditions, including headache." Given the obvious health benefits of exercise, a program of aerobic exercise is certainly warranted for people who suffer from headache. As usual, make sure you are evaluated and cleared by a healthcare professional, should you decide to begin a new exercise program.

There is limited literature on exercise for cervicogenic headache: one randomized, multicenter, controlled trial from Australia has investigated aerobic exercise. In 2000, these researchers from the University of Queensland found that, in the fifty individuals who exercised, there was a significant reduction in neck pain as well as in headache intensity and duration. It is equally impressive that these results persisted throughout the twelve-month follow-up period.

Acupuncture, PENS, and TENS for Migraine and Tension Headaches

Over 2,000 years old, acupuncture has been used by the Chinese to treat virtually every medical condition known. Acupuncture employs strategically placed needles in "points" that are alleged to balance yin and yang and restore health by increasing energy flow through "channels." Sometimes, a small electric current is passed through the acupuncture needle to enhance this effect. A complete discussion of this rich form of traditional Chinese medicine is beyond the scope of this book. There are, however, about 365 specific acupuncture points, with several thousand additional points located on the hands, head, and ears. In the West, acupuncture is used for treating chronic pain and alcohol and drug abuse. How acupuncture works has remained a subject of extreme controversy for decades. Recent research, however, has shed new light on how this ancient practice offers benefit. According to a Harvard researcher, acupuncture redistributes blood flow in the brain, possibly cutting off flow to pain-modulating centers.

Multiple studies have examined the beneficial

Acupuncture
An ancient Chinese medical system that employs the strategic placement of small needles just beneath the skin, and is successfully used to treat many pain syndromes.

effects of acupuncture on migraine. In one early study, it was reported that 81 percent of those who suffered from "chronic headaches" experienced improved symptoms following acupuncture. Another trial in Austria performed acupuncture on twenty-six patients with chronic migraines. Following treatment, 69 percent of the patients reported improved symptoms; 58 percent of the participants maintained improvement at three years. The authors also found that medication use decreased by 50 percent.

Another randomized, controlled clinical trial compared metoprolol with acupuncture in eighty-five people with migraine. According to the study, published in the *Journal of Internal Medicine* in 1994, acupuncture was "equipotent to metoprolol in the influence on frequency and duration (but not severity) of attacks, and superior in terms of negative side-effects." Even more impressive, a

Metoprolol
A beta-blocker drug that is used in the pharmaceutical treatment of migraine.

randomized, controlled clinical trial compared acupuncture versus flunarizine in 160 women with migraine. According to the report, acupuncture was able to "significantly lower the number of migraine attacks at two and four months of therapy when compared to flunarizine; however, after six months, these differences disappeared. Less use of migraine medication was also observed in the acupuncture group. The authors concluded, "acupuncture proved to be adequate for migraine prophylaxis. Relative to flunarizine, acupuncture treatment exhibited greater effectiveness in the first months of therapy and superior tolerability. A trial published in 2003 found that acupuncture was superior to TENS (transcutaneous electrical nerve stimulation) and laser therapy for reducing migraine-attack frequency.

Acupuncture has also been evaluated for the treatment of acute migraine attacks. One randomized, controlled multicenter study from Germany, by D. Melchart, et al., in 2003, reported that "a full migraine attack was prevented in 21 of 60 (35 percent) patients receiving acupuncture." While there exists substantial literature on acupuncture for migraine, studies on acupuncture for tension headache are more elusive. In a study of forty-one patients with migraine and muscle-tension headache, more than 50 percent of the participants reported improved symptoms following acupuncture, with nine patients having "very marked" relief. Another study, published in the *American Journal of Chinese Medicine*, reported that acupuncture was effective at relieving tension-headache symptoms. A recent study in sixty-nine individuals from Germany found "a significant but weak improvement" for tension headache treated with acupuncture.

Finally, percutaneous electrical nerve stimulation (PENS) employs a small electric current that is passed through needles placed in strategic bodily locations, kind of like jazzed up acupuncture. There are two studies that have examined PENS for headache. One study from the Eugene McDermott Center for Pain Management in Dallas used PENS to treat thirty patients with tension, migraine, or posttraumatic headache. The authors, Ahmed, et al., found that PENS was superior to needles alone when used for two weeks, three times weekly for thirty minutes. According to the article, pain scores decreased in tension, migraine, and posttraumatic headache by 58 percent, 59 percent, and 52 percent, respectively. Similar improvements in sleep quality and physical activity were also noted. The other study is a case report of PENS that was used successfully to prevent migraine following electroconvulsive therapy.

Another electrical stimulation technique used to treat pain is transcutaneous electrical nerve stimulation (TENS). TENS employs a small electric current applied to the skin, which ultimately enters the muscles. While TENS is commonly used to treat back pain, there is only one study on TENS for migraine. This randomized controlled clinical study published in 2003 found that two weeks of TENS significantly decreased the number of migraine days in the twenty women treated. Additional studies are needed; however, since TENS and PENS are low-risk procedures, a trial may be attempted in those who have not had success with other therapies.

Biofeedback for Tension and Migraine Headaches

Biofeedback trains individuals to exert control over bodily functions like breathing and blood pressure. This training appears to be especially useful in medical conditions in which psychological factors play a significant role. Biofeedback is successfully used in the treatment of chronic pain, anxiety, insomnia, and asthma. It is especially popular for treating children with headache, given its virtually nonexistent side-effect profile compared to the potential side effects of traditional headache medications.

Biofeedback
A form of alternative therapy aimed at achieving increased mastery over autonomic bodily functions, and often used to control stress as well as to treat headache.

Several trials have investigated the impact of electromyographic (EMG) biofeedback for tension headache. One study by L. Grazzi, et al., in 2001, examined thirty-eight juveniles over a three-year period. According to the authors "headaches improved measurably immediately following treatment, with further gains being evident through three years." Another randomized, controlled clinical trial in 1995 from the Biofeedback and Psychophysiological Disorders

Clinic in Georgia compared the efficacy of three biofeedback techniques: standard twelve-session frontal EMG biofeedback, twelve-session upper-trapezius EMG biofeedback, and standard seven-session progressive muscle relaxation therapy. Headache frequency was reduced in all three groups, with 100 percent of the trapezius group reporting reduced headaches. Finally, a 1991 study in tension headache using EMG biofeedback found that one-half of the subjects experienced a 50 percent or greater reduction in headache frequency. The authors noted that biofeedback increased the number of headache-free days, reduced peak headache activity, and reduced medication use.

Biofeedback has also been investigated for migraine headaches. In one randomized, controlled clinical study from the University of Alabama, thirty children were treated with biofeedback. Not only did "headache frequency and duration" improve, but at six months, 80 percent of the biofeedback group were symptom free. In another trial, thirty-two children with migraine were given "relaxation training, temperature biofeedback, and cognitive training." Forty-five percent of the children experienced improvement that was maintained during the seven-month follow-up. According to the authors, this improvement resulted from "a decrease in state anxiety and an increase in the ability to relax." Similar findings are observed for adults with migraine; one study reported "significant reductions in pain, depression, and anxiety."

Finally, a 1992 study examined thirty-four patients with chronic headaches, comparing autogenic relaxation therapy electromyographic (EMG) biofeedback to autogenic relaxation therapy/temperature biofeedback. While both techniques proved effective, relaxation with EMG biofeedback was reported as superior.

Chiropractic for Migraine, Tension, and Cervicogenic Headache

Chiropractic is based on the premise that the alignment of joints and muscles with each other and with the spine influence health. Chiropractors attempt to influence health and disease by manual manipulation of these structures. Indeed, people who suffer from musculoskeletal pain as well as headache often benefit from chiropractic manipulation. One of the reasons why chiropractic manipulation works in migraine and tension headaches is that both of these syndromes are associated with spinal and musculoskeletal dysfunction.

Several studies have examined the impact of chiropractic manipulation on headache. One randomized, controlled clinical study from Australia reported that "migraine frequency, duration, disability, and medication use" decreased significantly following spinal manipulation. Equally impressive, 22 percent of the study subjects reported a 90 percent reduction in migraine following two months of therapy. Another trial compared spinal manipulation to amitriptyline for migraines. This study found that during active treatment amitriptyline resulted in a 49 percent decrease in headache scores compared to 40 percent for the spinal manipulation; however, "during the posttreatment follow-up period, the reduction from baseline was 24% for amitriptyline, 42% for spinal manipulation."

Amitriptyline
An antidepressant sometimes used in the treatment of migraine.

While data is limited, studies also suggest that manipulation can help tension headaches. One randomized, controlled clinical trial from the Northwestern College of Chiropractic compared spinal manipulation with amitriptyline for tension headache. These researchers found that in the spinal manipulation group, 32 percent had less intense headaches, 42 percent had reduced headache frequency, and 30 percent indicated less medication use. Surprisingly, the amitriptyline group did not improve and some participants even had a "slight worsening" of symptoms. In addition, 82.1 percent of the amitriptyline group had side effects compared to 4.3 percent in the spinal manipulation group. The authors went on to report that "the patients who received spinal manipulative therapy experienced a sustained therapeutic benefit in all major outcomes in contrast to the patients that received amitriptyline therapy, who reverted to baseline." While further research will be needed to confirm these findings, this study clearly gives a ringing endorsement to manipulation for tension headache. Admittedly, these results are encouraging; however, not all studies have demonstrated positive findings. For instance, one randomized, controlled clinical trial on spinal manipulation for episodic tension headache found that this treatment "does not seem to have a positive effect on episodic tension-type headache." The jury may still be out on manipulation for tension headache; nevertheless, given the limited positive data, a trial is certainly worth considering.

Finally, several studies examine spinal manipulation for cervicogenic headache. One randomized, controlled clinical trial enrolled twenty-eight individuals who received "high-velocity, low-amplitude cervical manipulation twice a week for 3 weeks." These researchers found that with cervical manipulation, medication use dropped by 36 percent, the "number of headache hours per day" fell by 69 percent, and headache intensity was reduced 36 percent. The authors concluded that "spinal manipulation has a significant positive effect in cases of cervicogenic headache. In 2002,

Cervicogenic Headache

Similar to tension headache, these headaches arise from cervical musculoskeletal dysfunction.

another randomized, multicenter, controlled trial from Australia investigated manipulative therapy in fifty individuals with cervicogenic headache. These researchers from the University of Queensland found that manipulative therapy produced a significant reduction in neck pain as well as headache intensity and duration. Furthermore, these findings persisted through the twelve-month follow-up period.

For most people, chiropractic treatment is relatively safe with the most common side effects being fatigue, headache, pain, and discomfort in the treatment area. Spinal manipulation, however, does carry the risk of rare vascular dissection. Vascular dissection occurs when an artery splits lengthwise, resulting in a partial tear of the vessel. Symptoms range from none to headache to stroke: a very serious and life-threatening complication. Hence, the use of spinal manipulation for headache must be approached with extreme caution. Despite the existence of favorable reports, given the potential complications of spinal manipulation, I would only recommend its use as a last resort.

Massage Therapy for Migraine and Tension Headaches

Massage therapy employs massage or touch to various bodily regions to promote relaxation or to relieve stress or pain or both. Several researchers have successfully explored the impact of massage therapy in tension headache. In 1990, K. Puustjarvi, et al., followed twenty-one people who had chronic tension headache while they underwent six months of deep tissue upper-body massage. During the treatment period, these people experienced increased range of motion in their neck with decreased pain scores. Likewise, the number of days with pain decreased significantly. The authors concluded "this study confirmed clinical and physiological effects of massage." A study in 2002 from the Boulder Colorado College of Massage Therapy reported that massage decreased the frequency and duration of tension headache.

Posture Education
Instructions in the proper way to sit, stand, and so on, as well as identification of postures that may be related to health problems.

Massage therapy appears to be especially effective when combined with other treatments. For instance, one study in 1996 from the Mercy Medical Center enrolled twenty patients into a three-week period of posture education, isotonic exercise, massage, and neck stretching. These researchers found that not only were there significant improvements in headache symptoms, but these benefits lasted for over a year.

Data also exists regarding massage for migraine. A 1997 trial by K. R. Wylie, et al., found that massage/relaxation therapy resulted in a "significant improvement in pain ratings." Another case report described the prevention of a migraine by massage of the superficial temporal arteries.

As usual, the best treatment for migraine, and for almost any medical condition, is a multidisciplinary approach. Indeed, a group of researchers from Canada studied a program of exercise, stress management, diet, and massage therapy in forty-one patients with migraine. According to their report, following treatment, these individuals experienced statistically significant positive changes in "pain frequency, pain intensity, pain duration, functional status, quality of life, health status, pain related disability, and depression"— changes that persisted during the three-month follow-up period. Given these findings and the low-risk profile of massage therapy, this modality is highly recommended for anyone who suffers from headaches.

Physical Therapy for Tension Headache

Using a variety of touch, exercise, and stretching techniques, physical therapy can treat a wide range of conditions from stroke to headache to posttraumatic rehabilitation. While there is limited data on physical therapy for headache, from the available literature, it appears that this treatment may work. This is especially true if physical therapy is combined with other treatments such as biofeedback. For instance, one study from the Mercy Medical Center enrolled twenty patients into a three-week period of posture education, isotonic exercise, massage, and neck stretching. These researchers reported significant improvement in headache symptoms that lasted for over a year. Another study from the University of Pittsburgh Medical Center in 1998 reported improved headache symptoms in 14 percent of those who had physical therapy alone compared with 47 percent of participants who combined physical therapy with relaxation training and thermal biofeedback. Reviewing the literature, it appears that a trial of physical therapy combined with another treatment technique may be of value in helping relieve headache pain.

Reflexology for Tension and Migraine Headaches

Reflexology employs the manipulation of bodily pressure points to relieve pain and improve health. One study examined reflexology in 220 individuals with tension and migraine headaches for six months. At three months, the authors found that 81 percent of the participants "reported that they were helped by the treatments or were cured of their headache problems." Nineteen percent were able to stop medication use. Further studies will be needed regarding reflexology for headache; however, given these encouraging initial results along with the low side-effect profile of this therapy, reflexology is worthy of consideration.

Headache Support Groups

Having headaches can be hard, and it may be helpful to talk to people who share your problem. Several headache support groups and on-line resources are available for adults and children with headaches. An excellent on-line resource that offers a state-by-state listing of headache support groups can be found at www.headaches.org/consumer/supportgroups.html. An extensive database of headache-related information is sponsored by the American Council for Headache Education (ACHE). ACHE was founded in 1990 and its website can be visited at www.achenet.org. For those wishing to have an on-line headache support group experience, a great site that offers information as well as support group chats can be visited at www.headachesupportgroups.com/aboutus.htm.

CHAPTER 5

HEADACHE DRUGS

Despite our best efforts, there will always be people who will need medication to control their headaches. Of all the headache therapies discussed so far, it is the pharmacologic interventions that have consistently demonstrated the greatest efficacy for the most people. Without question, the best offense is a good defense and the removal of triggers, when identified, is the most important intervention you can make when it comes to headaches. Drugs are certainly not the best way to treat any medical condition; however, for some people, medications will remain an occasional, and at times a permanent, fact of life.

There is no doubt that drugs can cause problems of their own and that headache agents are notorious for side effects. What I find disturbing, however, is when authors slander headache medications, calling them poisons and accusing them of doing more harm than good. While it is true that many medications have potentially disturbing side effects, and true that some physicians rely too heavily on medications to treat head pain, it is also true that there are millions of people whose lives have been dramatically improved by these agents.

Nevertheless, one of the most common problems with the use of pharmaceuticals for the treatment of headache, especially chronic headache, is that these agents can actually cause headaches. Known as "analgesic rebound headache" or "medication overuse headache," this syndrome can occur in a person who habitually takes medication to treat headache. Once the medication is withdrawn, this person experiences a headache as a result of discontinuing the medication, thereby necessitating more frequent drug use. Thus begins a vicious cycle of headache followed by chronic medication use, which leads to this syndrome. As a physician, I have treated many people who have this habitual pattern of drug use. Indeed, the only way to treat this condition is to convince the individual to totally abstain from medication use for a week and see if the headaches recur or go away—an admittedly unpleasant but necessary experience.

So knowledge is power, and the more you know about the medicines you take, the more effective they become. While the purpose of this book is to get you medication free or dramatically reduce the amount of medication you are taking, the purpose of this chapter is to enlighten you about the side effects of headache medications while extracting the most benefit. When used properly, drugs can be good for you. Indeed, while most of these agents, when used properly, are safe and effective, some have a reputation for unpleasant and potentially lethal side effects, ranging from sedation to dangerous cardiac heart rhythms. For the majority of headache sufferers, however, the most disturbing side effects are the sedation and fatigue, which can be particularly devastating.

With respect to migraine, the basic tenet of drug therapy is to control the symptoms with as few drugs as possible. Depending on the severity of the symptoms, one drug may be used or many drugs may be used. Doctors typically start with one drug and add additional agents as needed. Once symptoms demonstrate stable improvement, many physicians will slowly withdraw therapy to reduce the patient's drug use as much as possible. Indeed, following effective therapy, some people are able to remain drug free for a period of time, their symptoms greatly improve, and they have fewer and less severe attacks.

People with mild headache symptoms usually respond well to oral therapy, whereas those who have severe symptoms may need injections or intravenous agents. While multiple agents are used to treat headaches, the three major drug classes are anti-inflammatories, serotonin agonists, and dopamine antagonists. Like most medical conditions, what works for one individual may not work for another, and a certain amount of trial and error is needed to find the right products. Headache treatment needs to be individualized, and you should expect your healthcare provider to take the time to find out what is wrong and what works and does not work. Some people will achieve effective relief with one agent, whereas others may try multiple drugs in different combinations with only modest results.

With respect to migraine, if you must take medication, it is important that you do so under the guidance of an experience healthcare professional. In general, migraine medication should be taken at the beginning of an attack, and the dosage increased if the attack does not respond to initial therapy. What follows is a brief review of the typical agents used for headache along with their pluses and minuses.

Acetaminophen

Acetaminophen is the active ingredient commonly found in medications like Tylenol. When used properly, acetaminophen is a relatively safe and effective drug. Because acetaminophen is so common, people often wrongly assume that it does not have potentially serious side effects. The most serious side effect of acetaminophen is liver damage, which can be fatal. It normally takes a significant and intentional overdose of acetaminophen to cause liver damage; however, people with liver disease are at risk of acetaminophen-induced liver damage, even with modest use.

Although public awareness regarding acetaminophen-related liver toxicity has increased thanks to heightened publicity, it may surprise many people to learn that acetaminophen can also damage the kidneys, if used improperly. Acetaminophen also has multiple drug interactions. Similar to aspirin, people who are taking blood thinners should not take acetaminophen. Likewise, acetaminophen should not be used with alcohol and has history of interacting with anti-seizure medications. Nevertheless, when used properly, acetaminophen can safely help relieve headache symptoms. Acetaminophen production also blocks cyclooxygenase and prostaglandin, two chemicals known to mediate pain.

Dosage

The typical acetaminophen dose is 325–650 milligrams every four hours, not to exceed 4 grams daily.

Aspirin

An old drug, aspirin has been used for decades to help relieve all sorts of pain as well as fever. Aspirin works by decreasing the synthesis of prostaglandin, a chemical involved in mediating pain pathways. In fever, aspirin acts on the hypothalamus, helping to normalize body temperature. The public perception of aspirin is similar to that of acetaminophen, and many people assume that, because aspirin is so common, it must be safe. Although most people who take aspirin suffer no ill effects, this drug can cause stomach upset, occasionally accompanied by dangerous internal bleeding. Other uncommon side effects include reduced white blood cells and platelets. White blood cells are important for fighting infection, and platelets are needed to help blood clot and help control bleeding. This is why some people who take aspirin bruise easily. It's also why aspirin should not be used in people who are taking blood thinners, such as warfarin.

Other negative aspirin-related drug interactions include alcohol, ACE inhibitors, and anti-seizure agents. Aspirin should never be given to child who has flulike symptoms, as this can precipitate Reye's syndrome.

Reye's Syndrome

An illness that occurs in children under the age of fifteen and is characterized by liver damage, vomiting, and central nervous system damage.

Dosage

The typical aspirin dose is 325–650 milligrams every four hours. Never take more than 4 grams of aspirin daily. A particularly potent combination is acetaminophen, aspirin, and caffeine; it is effective even in moderately severe migraine attacks.

Muscle Relaxants

Muscle relaxants are occasionally used in tension headache, when muscular dysfunction has been documented. The chief drawback to muscle relaxants is their sedating effect, especially when used with alcohol. Other uncommon side effects include abnormal heart rhythms, dry mouth, and urinary retention. For these reasons, muscle relaxants should not be used in the elderly or in people with heart disease.

Nonsteroidal Anti-inflammatory Drugs (NSAIDs)

NSAIDs have emerged as one of the primary drugs for headache pain. The most common NSAID is ibuprofen, a drug found in a bewildering array of over-the-counter and prescription agents. NSAIDs are not only potent analgesics but also display anti-inflammatory action and are commonly used in arthritis. Similar to aspirin, NSAIDs reduce pain by blocking prostaglandin synthesis, a major chemical pain mediator.

The chief drawback of NSAIDs is their potential to cause stomach irritation as well as gastrointestinal bleeding. This notorious feature of NSAIDs is a common cause of stomach ulcers as well as hospital admission for internal bleeding. As with many pain medications, NSAIDs can increase the risk of bleeding and should not be taken with blood thinners. NSAIDs can also interact with blood pressure agents, diuretics, and digoxin. When used properly, NSAIDs can offer effective headache relief. NSAIDs work best when taken early in an attack; however, efficacy declines with increasing attack severity.

Dosage

For ibuprofen, the typical dose is 200–800 milligrams every six hours. Do not take more than 3.2 grams of ibuprofen daily.

Serotonin Agonists

As you learned earlier, serotonin dysfunction is implicated in migraine, and agents that act on serotonin receptors can relieve migraine symptoms. The older serotonin agonists, such as ergotamine and dihydroergotamine, nonselectively stimulated several serotonin receptors and this occasionally resulted in nausea. Several different types of serotonin receptors exist; however, only a few are believed to participate in migraine attacks. While the older, nonselective serotonin agonists have some drawbacks compared with newer more selective agents like the triptans, headache recurrence appears to be less of a problem with older agents, such as ergotamine. Ergotamine has also

Agonist
An agent that promotes or stimulates a chemical, biochemical, or hormone-mediated reaction.

been successfully used for treating cluster headaches. A potential problem with daily use of ergotamine is ergotism, and this side effect restricts the amount of ergotamine that can be taken weekly.

Ergotism
A complex and dangerous condition that can result in vascular and neurological dysfunction.

Newer agents, such as the triptan drugs, are called selective serotonin agonists and have a cleaner mechanism of action in that they only interact with certain types of serotonin receptors. The triptans (for example, rizatriptan, sumatriptan, and zolmitriptan) represent a new headache drug class and are primarily used to treat migraine. They take advantage of the fact that serotonin-related abnormalities are observed in patients with migraine. Triptans stimulate a sub-class of serotonin-related receptors that are found on nerves and blood vessels, and so achieve their antimigraine effects.

The triptans are virtually equally effective, although rizatriptan is shorter acting and perhaps more effective. Quick action is important for pain control, and in general, the more rapid the action the better the results. The fastest-acting serotonin agonists are nasal preparations, such as dihydroergotamine and sumatriptan. These drugs are easy to use and offer rapid action. However, they taste awful, and some people have experienced dosing problems with them. In part because of these complications, nasal sprays for migraine only work in about half the population. Serotonin agonists like dihydroergotamine and sumatriptan can also be given as a subcutaneous injections. Agents that can be injected appear to demonstrate the greatest results and are effective in about 80 percent of those who use them.

While triptans are effective, up to 90 percent of patients have side effects, which tend to be mild and short-lived. Another drawback is that some patients have to take another drug with the triptan for adequate relief. A major problem with the triptans is that the headaches tend to recur. Although these shortcomings are not seen in all patients, they do limit the use of triptans as single-agent therapy. Finally, triptans should not be used by people who have heart disease.

Dopamine-Receptor Antagonists

Dopamine-receptor antagonists, such as metoclopramide and prochlorperazine, are typically used in the treatment of migraine and are often given with another drug. As you learned in Chapter 2, dopamine stimulation can induce migrainelike symptoms, and drugs that antagonize dopamine have been developed for treating migraine. Dopamine-receptor antagonists are typically given with another antimigraine agent, so they can act together.

Antagonist
An agent that inhibits or prevents a chemical, biochemical, or hormone-mediated reaction.

An important beneficial feature of the dopamine-receptor antagonists is that they reduce nausea and vomiting. Equally important, these agents help normalize stomach motion. Abnormal gastric motility is seen in migraine and can impair medication absorption. The major drawback to the dopamine-receptor antagonists is their side effects, which can be debilitating, severe, and potentially life threatening. Indeed, there is an extensive list of side effects associated with these agents, which includes seizures, blood abnormalities, hallucinations, dizziness, and fatigue. Hypersensitivity to dopamine is another potential side effect that is described in individuals who have genetic abnormalities in dopamine receptors.

Caffeine for Migraine and Tension Headaches

Is caffeine a drug or a natural remedy? Clearly this is a matter of opinion; however, caffeine has been successfully used in the treatment of tension and migraine headaches and is commonly found in many prescription and over-the-counter medications. Caffeine is also seen in many foods, such as chocolate and soft drinks. Indeed, many people who suffer from migraine will tell you that several cups of coffee provide relief. Multiple studies have documented the efficacy of caffeine either alone or in combination with another agent for tension and migraine headaches. While there are health risks associated with excessive caffeine ingestion, caffeine is clearly an effective, inexpensive, and readily available remedy for many people with headache.

On the flip side, some people actually have their headaches triggered by caffeine. Hence, caffeine may be either helping or causing your headaches. Most people who regularly ingest caffeinated beverages will know if caffeine helps or hurts. If there is any doubt regarding how you react, I suggest a caffeine-free trial to determine if your headaches get better or worse. If you are a regular caffeine user, you can expect to get a headache simply from caffeine withdrawal. Given the complexities of caffeine ingestion and how this agent relates to headaches, if you are uncertain as to how caffeine is affecting your headaches, you should seek consultation with a healthcare professional, who can help guide you in determining if caffeine is a friend or foe.

Butorphanol and Narcotics

Butorphanol is a nasal agent, otherwise known as Stadol (its trade name) and is used to treat pain; its use is limited because it is a narcotic. Narcotics are the strongest pain relievers and come in several types. The major problem with narcotics is that they can be addictive and can cause multiple side effects, such as sedation and constipation. The use of narcotics, such as hydrocodone

(Vicoden) or oxycodone (Percodan), can be especially problematic, because withdrawal from these agents can produce headaches that can be difficult to distinguish from migraine.

Prophylactic Migraine Therapy

For people who suffer at least three migraine attacks monthly, the use of prophylactic (preventative) medication should be strongly considered. The major drawback to prophylactic therapy is that the medication must be taken daily, and the results are not seen for up to six weeks. A number of agents are available for prophylactic therapy and include tricyclic antidepressants, antiseizure medications, beta-blockers, serotonin-related agents, and occasionally, monoamine oxidase inhibitors (MAOIs). MAOIs are rarely, if ever, used today as they have multiple drug interactions and react with foods that contain tyramine.

Conclusion

I hope this book has helped you learn about headaches and how to prevent and treat them. As you have seen, there are many different types of headaches, and they can range from a mild annoyance to a severe and repetitive, debilitating event. While the vast majority of headaches are benign, I hope you have learned a little about how to distinguish between a common migraine or tension headache and something more serious. Mercifully, most headaches are benign and, indeed, preventable. Look closely at headaches in the context of your life and lifestyle. Do you notice your symptoms occur after eating certain foods or experiencing stressful events? If so, try to remove these foods from your diet. If stress is a major headache trigger, do your best to minimize the stress in your life. I realize this may be easier said than done in a high-stress world; however, reducing stress is a win-win situation for everyone. If reducing stress is not practical, strongly consider some of the alternative therapies outlined in Chapter 4, such as exercise or biofeedback, that can not only help headaches but also reduce stress.

If simple lifestyle modification does not work, consider the use of supplements, a subject we explored extensively in Chapter 3. Some trial and error may be involved in finding the right supplement; however, most people can find one or two that work. Finding the right supplement may be a bit more involved for people who suffer from severe headaches. People who have severe head pain may have to use more than one supplement; however, even people who have severe symptoms can achieve benefit. Equally important is to combine the use of supplements with an alternative therapy like exercise or acupuncture: methods that can work synergistically in helping to relieve your symptoms. As with most medical problems, pharmacotherapy, as discussed in Chapter 5, is another treatment avenue; however, the use of drugs, while clearly indicated in certain individuals, should be the therapy of last resort. Also, seek to develop a trusting relationship with a healthcare professional who can help guide you through the various therapies.

Perhaps the most important take-home message is that for many people headache symptoms do not have to control your life and are preventable. Indeed, many headaches are precipitated by stress, foods, or allergies. Identifying and removing these triggers is a critical step in achieving headache relief. Take control of your headaches— don't allow your headaches to take control of you! Much of the advice in this book can be used to make your home and life healthier. While a proper diet coupled with the judicious use of supplements can help you add healthy years to your life, it is equally important to live healthy. What I mean by "living healthy" is embracing a program of a healthy diet, adequate sleep, regular exercise, and a balanced positive outlook toward life that will enable you to enjoy many active and trouble-free decades. Although many headaches occur on their own, a significant percentage of headaches result from known triggers. Headaches do not occur in a vacuum; rather, for many of us, they are triggered by events that are part of our everyday life. It is your mission to identify these triggers and remove them from your life and home. Headaches are a part of life and to beat headaches we have to learn once again how to live. Learn to control your life and embrace a daily program of healthy living. Remove those triggers that are causing you misery, and you will not only overcome your headaches but also become the master of your own destiny.

SELECTED
REFERENCES

Ahmed, H. E., P. F. White, W. F. Craig, et al. Use of percutaneous electrical nerve stimulation (PENS) in the short-term management of headache. *Headache.* 2000; 40: 311–315.

Allais, G., C. De Lorenzo, P. E. Quirico, et al. Acupuncture in the prophylactic treatment of migraine without aura: A comparison with flunarizine. *Headache.* 2002; 42: 855–861.

Arena, J. G., G. M. Bruno, S. L. Hannah, et al. A comparison of frontal electromyographic biofeedback training, trapezius electromyographic biofeedback training, and progressive muscle relaxation therapy in the treatment of tension headache. *Headache.* 1995; 35: 411–419.

Boline, P. D., K. Kassak, G. Bronfort, et al. Spinal manipulation vs. amitriptyline for the treatment of chronic tension-type headaches: A randomized clinical trial. *J Manipulative Physiol Ther.* 1995; 18: 148–154.

Bove, G. and N. Nilsson. Spinal manipulation in the treatment of episodic tension-type headache: A randomized controlled trial. *JAMA.* 1998; 280: 1576–1579.

Diamond, S., F. Freitag, and S. B. Phillips, et al. Intranasal civamide for the acute treatment of migraine headache. *Cephalalgia.* 2000; 20: 597–602.

Ernst, E. and M. H. Pittler. The efficacy and safety of feverfew (*Tanacetum Parthenium* L.): an update of a systematic review. *Public Health Nutr.* 2000; 3: 509–514.

Gatto, G., D. Caleri, S. Michelacci, et al. Analgesizing effect of a methyl donor (S-adenosylmethionine) in migraine: An open clinical trial. *Int J Clin Pharmacol Res.* 1986; 6: 15–617.

Gobel, H., J. Fresenius, A. Heinze, et al. Effectiveness

of Oleum menthae piperitae and paracetamol in therapy of headache of the tension type. *Nervenarzt.* 1996; 67: 672–681.

Grazzi, L., F. Andrasik, D. D'Amico, et al. Electromyographic biofeedback-assisted relaxation training in juvenile episodic tension-type headache: Clinical outcome at three-year follow-up. *Cephalalgia.* 2001; 21: 798–803.

Hasselmark, L., R. Malmgren, and J. Hannerz. Effect of a carbohydrate-rich diet, low in protein-tryptophan, in classic and common migraine. *Cephalalgia.* 1987; 7: 87–92.

Hesse, J., B. Mogelvang, and H. Simonsen. Acupuncture versus metoprolol in migraine prophylaxis: A randomized trial of trigger point inactivation. *J Intern Med.* 1994; 235: 451–456.

Jull, G., P. Trott, H. Potter, et al. A randomized controlled trial of exercise and manipulative therapy for cervicogenic headache. *Spine.* 2002; 27: 1835–1843.

Launso, L., E. Brendstrup, and S. Arnber. An exploratory study of reflexological treatment for headache. *Altern Ther Health Med.* 1999; 5: 57–65.

Lemstra, M., B. Stewart, and W. P. Olszynski. Effectiveness of multidisciplinary intervention in the treatment of migraine: A randomized clinical trial. *Headache.* 2002; 42: 845–854.

Maissen, C. P. and H. P. Ludin. Comparison of the effect of 5-hydroxytryptophan and propranolol in the interval treatment of migraine. *Schweiz Med Wochenschr.* 1991; 121: 1585–1590.

Marks, D. R., A. Rapoport, D. Padla, et al. A double-blind placebo-controlled trial of intranasal capsaicin for cluster headache. *Cephalalgia.* 1993; 13: 114–116.

Mauskop, A. Alternative therapies in headache. Is there a role? *Med Clin North Am.* 2001; 85: 1077–1084.

Mauskop, A. and B. M. Altura. Role of magnesium in the pathogenesis and treatment of migraines. *Clin Neurosci.* 1998; 5: 24–27.

Melchart, D., J. Thormaehlen, S. Hager, et al. Acupuncture versus placebo versus sumatriptan for early treatment of migraine attacks: A randomized controlled trial. *J Intern Med.* 2003; 253: 181–188.

Narin, S. O., L. Pinar, D. Erbas, et al. The effects of exercise and exercise-related changes in blood nitrous oxide level on migraine headache. *Clin Rehabil.* 2003; 17: 624–630.

Nelson, C. F., G. Bronfort, R. Evans, et al. The efficacy of spinal manipulation, amitriptyline and the combination of both therapies for the prophylaxis of migraine headache. *J Manipulative Physiol Ther.* 1998; 21: 511–559.

Osterhaus, S. O., J. Passchier, H. van der Helm-Hylkema, et al. Effects of behavioral psychophysiological treatment on schoolchildren with migraine in a non-clinical setting: Predictors and process variables. *J Pediatr Psychol.* 1993;18:697–715.

Peres, M. F. and T. D. Rozen. Melatonin in the preventative treatment of chronic cluster headache. *Cephalalgia.* 2001; 21: 993–995.

Pfaffenrath, V., H. C. Diener, M. Fischer, et al. The efficacy and safety of Tanacetum Parthenium (feverfew) in migraine prophylaxis—a double-blind, multicenter, randomized placebo-controlled dose-response study. *Cephalalgia.* 2002; 22: 523–532.

Pittler, M. H., B. K. Vogler, and E. Ernst. Feverfew for preventing migraine. *Cochrane Database Syst Rev.* 2000; 3: CD002286.

Pradalier, A., P. Bakouche, G. Baudesson, et al. Failure of omega-3 polyunsaturated fatty acids in prevention of migraine: A double-blind study versus placebo. *Cephalalgia.* 2001; 21: 818–822.

Pringsheim, T., E. Magnoux, C. F. Dobson, et al. Melatonin as adjunctive therapy in the prophylaxis of cluster headache. *Headache.* 2002; 42: 787–792.

Quinn, C., C. Chandler, and A. Moraska. Massage therapy and frequency of chronic tension headaches. *Am J Public Health.* 2002; 92: 1657–1661.

Rozen, T. D., M. L. Oshinsky, C. A. Gebeline, et al. Open label trial of coenzyme Q_{10} as a migraine preventive. *Cephalalgia.* 2002; 22: 137–141.

Schoenen, J., J. Jacquy, and M. Lenaerts. Effectiveness of high-dose riboflavin in migraine prophylaxis. A randomized controlled trial. *Neurology.* 1998; 50: 466–470.

Thys-Jacobs, S. Vitamin D and calcium in menstrual migraine. *Headache.* 1994; 34: 544–546.

Titus, F., A. Davalos, J. Alom, et al. 5-Hydroxytryptophan versus methysergide in the prophylaxis of migraine. Randomized clinical trial. *Eur Neurol.* 1986; 25: 327–329.

Velling, D. A., D. W. Dodick, and J. J. Muir. Sustained-release niacin for prevention of migraine headache. *Mayo Clin Proc.* 2003; 78: 770–771.

OTHER BOOKS
AND RESOURCES

Bic, Z., F. Bic, and L. F. Bic. *No More Headaches, No More Migraines: A Proven Approach to Headaches and Migraines,* Avery Penguin Putnam, 1999.

Bucholz, D. and S. G. Reich. *Heal Your Headache: The 1-2-3 Program for Taking Charge of Your Pain,* New York: Workman, 2002.

Lang, S. and L. Robbers *Headache Help: A Complete Guide to Understanding Headaches and Medications That Relieve Them.* Boston: Houghton Mifflin, 2000.

Spierings, E. L. H. *Headache.* Butterworth-Heinemann, 1998

An extensive database of headache-related information is sponsored by the American Council for Headache Education (ACHE) and can be found at www.achenet.org.

GreatLife Magazine
Consumer magazine with articles on vitamins, minerals, herbs, and foods.
Available for free at many health and natural food stores.

Let's Live Magazine
Consumer magazine with emphasis on the health benefits of vitamins, minerals, and herbs.

Customer service:
1-800-676-4333
P.O. Box 74908
Los Angeles, CA 90004

Subscriptions: 12 issues per year, $19.95 in the U.S.; $31.95 outside the U.S.

Physical Magazine

Magazine oriented to body builders and other serious athletes.

Customer service:

1-800-676-4333

P.O. Box 74908

Los Angeles, CA 90004

Subscriptions: 12 issues per year, $19.95 in the U.S.; $31.95 outside the U.S.

The Nutrition Reporter™ newsletter

Monthly newsletter that summarizes recent medical research on vitamins, minerals, and herbs.

Customer service:

P.O. Box 30246

Tucson, AZ 85751-0246

e-mail: jack@thenutritionreporter.com

www.nutritionreporter.com

Subscriptions: 12 issues per year, $26 in the U.S.; $32 U.S. or $48 CNC for Canada; $38 for other countries.

INDEX